Trips for Those Over 50

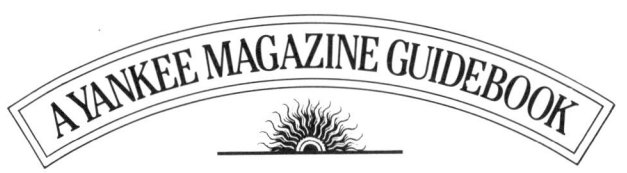

A YANKEE MAGAZINE GUIDEBOOK

TRIPS FOR THOSE OVER 50

By Harriet Webster

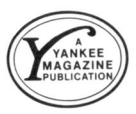

YANKEE BOOKS

A division of
Yankee Publishing Incorporated
Dublin, New Hampshire

For Doris, who's truly one of a kind.

Designed by Jill Shaffer

Yankee Publishing Incorporated
Dublin, New Hampshire 03444

First Edition
Copyright 1988 by Harriet Webster

Printed in the United States of America.
All rights reserved, including the right to reproduce
this book, or any parts thereof, in any form, except
for the inclusion of brief quotations in a review.

Library of Congress Cataloging-in-Publication Data
Webster, Harriet.
Trips for those over 50 / by Harriet Webster. — 1st ed.
p. cm.
Includes index.
ISBN 0-89909-158-X : $9.95
1. New England — Description and travel — 1981- — Guide-books
I. Title.
F2.3.W398   1988
917.4'0443—dc19   87-34550
CIP

Contents

Planning Your Travels 6

CONNECTICUT
Fairfield and Westport 15
The Northeast Corner 21
Route 7: Brookfield to Norfolk 28

RHODE ISLAND
Narragansett 34

MASSACHUSETTS
Sandwich 40
Boston 47
Salem 54
Rockport 63
Sheffield 71
Williamstown and North Adams 76

NEW HAMPSHIRE
Canterbury 84
Meredith 88
Franconia Notch 94
Franconia and Sugar Hill 100
Hanover 106

VERMONT
Route 30: Brattleboro to Townshend 112
Windsor 119
Weston 124
Middlebury 131
Shelburne 137
Burlington 144

MAINE
Freeport 150
Bath 156
Castine 161
Blue Hill 167

Index 173

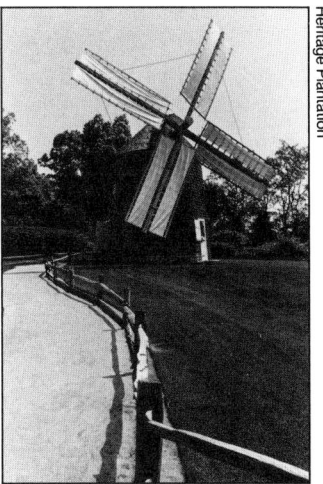

At The Old East Mill on Heritage Plantation in Sandwich, Massachusetts, they still grind corn the old-fashioned way.

Planning Your Travels

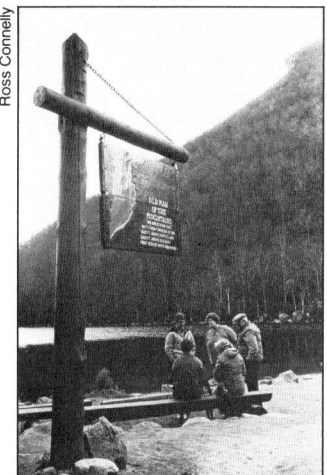

New Hampshire's Old Man of the Mountain watches over travelers paused for a rest on the shore of Profile Lake.

The very best trips are those that make a traveler feel comfortable and at ease and at the same time manage to brush away the cobwebs of everyday routine. Such trips deliver great satisfaction, both in the doing and in the remembering. They complement one's basic nature, expanding upon predictable pleasures and introducing new ones. New England is the perfect territory for staging such trips. Compact yet diverse, it boasts dramatic mountain scenery, gentle hills and valleys, and a coastline that ranges from rugged to serene. Well steeped in history and absolutely up-to-date in recreational, cultural, and academic opportunities, New England is a good friend to many types of travelers. We feel certain that you will come to share our enthusiasm as you become acquainted with our region.

When it comes to trip planning, you, as a mature traveler, have at least one advantage over your younger counterparts: You know yourself better. With a kaleidoscope of experiences stretching behind you, you're in tune with your own rhythms, tastes, and idiosyncrasies. You know that simply being away from home isn't going to change your need for an unhurried breakfast or the opportunity to take a good long walk in the evening. And that's the first ingredient for successful travels — in New England or anywhere else: knowing what kind of a person you are and what you need to be content.

This book is filled with vacation ideas specifically designed to appeal to older travelers. And because older travelers are hard to categorize — because some have more stamina than others; because some travel predominantly with spouse, many others with friends, and some individually; and most of all because interests among older travelers vary so widely — the trips outlined here cover many different subjects and lifestyles. We have tried to include both places where a couple can pursue their interests separately while vacationing together and places that are well suited to those who travel alone.

Why These Trips Are Recommended

The trips described in this book are based on our understanding that while mature travelers come in many guises, as a group you lean toward certain preferences. Many of you tell us that you prefer to visit places where you can use convenient local transportation to get from one attraction to another (try riding the trolley in Salem, Massachusetts) or to do your sightseeing (take a lake cruise or a scenic train ride from Meredith, New Hampshire). Still others have a penchant for a leisurely drive in the country, so we've included "shunpiker" excursions that will take you along the byways of The Northeast Corner in Connecticut, and Route 30: Brattleboro to Townshend in Vermont, to name just a couple possibilities. And because you tell us you like to avoid crowds and get the best value for your money, we've included ideas for off-season travel to popular summer destinations like Narragansett, Rhode Island.

For those who enjoy opportunities to recall experiences that hail back to childhood, we've listed trips that give you a chance to do such things as pick your own strawberries (Shelburne, Vermont), and attend an old-fashioned country auction (Sheffield, Massachusetts). We also recognize your enthusiasm for learning new things, your willingness to take the time to delve into subjects that you've never before had the time or opportunity to explore. To satisfy that need, we've described learning experiences that vary from afternoon workshops to full-time residential programs lasting several weeks.

Pace and Timing

The trips in this book are designed to blanket the six New England states. They include coastal towns and mountain villages, rural settings and urban centers. Some trips are best taken in summer, while others are most spectacular during fall foliage season. The trips vary in length from a day to a week or even longer. The choices you make will depend on your own tastes and concerns.

Some travelers thrive on a busy schedule. You like to be entertained, to take guided tours, to cover a lot of ground each day. Others favor a distinctly different pace. You don't like to be rushed, to have to adhere to a schedule. You prefer to plan your days according to how you feel when you wake up in the morning. Members of both groups will find many options in these pages.

Many older travelers have the opportunity to travel off-season, unrestricted by work and school schedules. To take advantage of your own flexibility, take into account other folks' inflexibility. That unhurried week of cross-country skiing you envision can turn into a nightmare if you inadvertently plan it for winter break, when many ski areas are packed to the gills with families. If you're in the market for a leisurely drive at peak foliage season, you'll find yourself unnecessarily frustrated by the traffic and crowds if you plan your trip for Columbus Day weekend.

In addition to the fact that you'll spend less time waiting in line at nonpeak times, it simply stands to reason that the people you meet — from waitresses to tour guides, shopkeepers to museum staffers — will be more congenial when they are less pressured. You'll be rewarded with more thoughtful and efficient service, and you'll find it easier to engage people in conversation.

Another benefit of a flexible schedule is that it can enable you to spend extra time when and where you want. If the idea of city sightseeing leaves you feeling exhausted and harried, even though you'd really like to visit the museums and take the time to explore the neighborhoods, go when you can spend four days instead of two. Rather than being frustrated by what you don't have the time or energy to see, you'll feel gratified by the luxury of being able to take your time, to quit for the day when you want, to explore unexpected places that turn up.

Be Careful about Assumptions

Don't assume that tickets will be available for the music festival the day you plan to attend. Call ahead to reserve so you aren't disappointed. Don't assume the rose garden will be in full bloom just because that's the way it's shown in the leaflet. If you want to see the roses at their glory, call ahead before leaving home; it may be a cold (and therefore late) growing season. If your cat is your trusty travel buddy, check ahead to be sure she'll be welcome where you plan to spend the night. Special diet? Call the restaurant in advance and find out whether they can accommodate you; if they can't, choose someplace else.

As a rule, the telephone can be your most useful tool when planning the specifics of your trip. Take this statement to heart, particularly when scheduling an outing that coincides with the beginning or end of the season noted in the ACCESS sections in this book. Places often adjust their start and finish dates according to the weather and a general sense of the business climate.

To Drive or Not to Drive

Most parts of New England are most easily reached by car. But that doesn't mean you have to be wedded to your vehicle. If you don't like to drive at night, try staying in a town where most of the evening activities are within walking distance of your hotel. Boston fits perfectly into this category. Or plan to stay at a hotel or inn like the Newfane Inn (see "Route 30: Brattleboro to Townshend," Vermont), which offers a pleasant restaurant where you can have a relaxed dinner before settling in for the evening. You might purposely choose a destination, like Rockport, Massachusetts, where you can walk to most of the places of interest, ignoring your car once you've arrived.

Traveling Solo

Our first words of advice: Do it! Don't miss out on a trip you really want to take just because you can't find a companion. Often you'll find that the same things that attract you to an area will attract others of similar interests. Traveling solo doesn't have to mean being lonely. One way to improve the chances of coming across congenial company is to enroll in a special interest workshop or trip. Sign up for a nature expedition sponsored by the Montshire Museum of Science or a craft workshop offered by the Hanover League of New Hampshire Craftsmen (see "Hanover," New Hampshire). The Silo and the Brookfield Craft Center (see "Route 7: Brookfield to Norfolk," Connecticut) conduct a year-round schedule of cooking and craft sessions, respectively. You'll meet other class participants, and in many cases you'll end up sharing meals with them. Enroll in an Elderhostel program (more about this in a moment) and you'll find yourself with dormmates as well as classmates. Traveling alone can give you great independence, and it doesn't have to mean being alone all the time, unless you prefer it that way.

Back to School

Think about becoming a full-time "on-campus" student again. Consider going to school to study what you truly *want* to study. "School" may be a residential session at the Fletcher Farm School for the Arts and Crafts (see "Weston," Vermont) or at the Haystack Mountain School of Crafts (see "Blue Hill," Maine), where the participants vary in age.

Or it may be formal courses offered by Elderhostel. Whether you want to delve into economic theory, brush up on your Italian, discuss Dostoyevsky over cocktails with your literature professor, or hone up on the ecology of the Maine wilderness, you'll find an Elderhostel program that will help you do it.

Programs run year-round and are open to anyone sixty years of age or older and the "student's" spouse. A participant who is at least sixty may be accompanied by a companion fifty years of age or older. It doesn't matter whether you have a Ph.D. or your formal education came to a screeching halt about the time you hit adolescence. Life experience and an openness to new ideas are what count.

Elderhostel programs run one week, and the all-inclusive fee covers room and board, tuition, extracurricular activities, and the use of many campus recreational and cultural facilities. Programs are based at colleges in each of the New England states, several of them within easy striking distance of the trips we outline in the pages that follow. Send for a complete catalog of course offerings, which is mailed for free three times a year. Write to Elderhostel, 80 Boylston Street, Suite 400, Boston, MA 02116.

Participation in an Elderhostel program provides an excellent focus for your vacation. You can explore the surrounding area in your free time while getting to know interesting people who share your enthusiasm for exploring new ideas. The Elderhostel academic environment is friendly and supportive. In most cases you'll live in a college dormitory and eat in the college commons in the company of fellow Elderhostelers. The catalog states: "You may express a single room preference when registering, but you must be willing to share a room in the event that no single accommodations are available. Bathroom facilities are generally shared." That's the hosteling element of Elderhostel, but don't let it put you off. Once you've read the catalog, you'll probably find that the programs are too tempting to ignore. All that's called for is a good dose of personal flexibility and enthusiasm for a new experience.

Saving Money

One of the best ways to stretch your travel dollars is to travel off-season and to avoid peak vacation periods. To do this most effectively, call ahead to inquire about special rates during certain periods. Also ask whether any package plans are available. In resort areas you can often stay three nights midweek for the same amount you'd pay for two nights on the weekend. In large cities, where hotels cater to business travelers, the opposite is true — the bargains are available on weekends.

When it comes to stretching your food dollars, one of the basic strategies is to have at least one "picnic" a day. Yours might take the form of take-out coffee and Danish for breakfast or deli sandwiches eaten in your room at night (particularly pleasant when you've had a long tiring day and would much rather curl up with a book or watch television than spend the evening in a restaurant). Or you might want to pack a classic picnic to eat by a waterfall or on a mountaintop. But whatever you choose, the basic idea is to avoid paying for three restaurant meals a day.

When you do eat out, if you find yourself continually served meals that are much too large, ask if it's acceptable to order from the children's menu or if reduced portions are available. Or ask if there is any objection to two people sharing an entrée. Leaving out the entrée and sticking to a soup-and-salad dinner or ordering two appetizers instead of a main course are also good strategies.

Another way to stretch your food dollars is to stay at an inn that includes breakfast in the room rate. Or you might look for a hotel that offers AP (American Plan) or MAP (Modified American Plan). AP rates include the cost of three meals a day. MAP includes the cost of two meals a day, usually breakfast and dinner. Again, it's best to ask ahead about such arrangements.

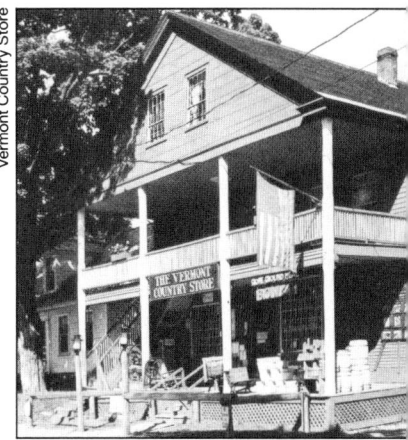

You can buy calico by the yard and candy by the piece at the Vermont Country Store in Weston.

Many establishments, from restaurants and hotels to transportation companies, theaters, and tourist attractions, offer discounts for senior citizens. The catch is that while many offer, few advertise. Even places that post their rates will seldom charge the senior citizen price unless you request it. But even if there is no sign, it makes sense to ask.

As you read the pages that follow, looking for trips that appeal to your tastes, be sure to consult the ACCESS section at the end of each chapter. Here you'll find mention of handicapped accessibility and senior discounts. In the Boston section you will see the notation "Golden Age Passport accepted." The Golden Age Passport is a free, lifetime entrance pass to all those national parks, monuments, historic sites, recreational areas, and national wildlife refuges administered by the federal government that charge entrance fees. To secure a pass, you need only be a United States citizen or permanent resident, sixty-two years of age or older. The passport provides free admission for both the permit holder and any other passengers in the same private noncommercial vehicle.

Passports must be obtained in person. They are issued at all national park system areas where entrance fees are charged, however, so it is not necessary to obtain the passport before starting your trip. You will need to bring along proof of age in the form of a driver's license, birth certificate, or Medicare card.

We hope that you will use the suggestions that follow to plan trips that complement your own tastes

How to Use the Chart

and needs. Most of all, we wish you pleasant, comfortable travels as you set about exploring New England, our special corner of the world.

The chart on page 13 provides a quick reference for the trips described in this book. Because all the trips (with the exception of Canterbury, New Hampshire) feature numerous places to visit, information in the chart refers to *all* the attractions included as part of a particular trip.

Most of the categories are self-explanatory. Further explanation of several categories is provided below.

Park/nature area refers to state and local parks, both public and private, and also includes wildlife sanctuaries.

"Old-fashioned" fun includes attractions such as old-fashioned carousel rides and pick-your-own fruit farms — places where you can still do things "the way they used to."

Water sports include canoeing, fishing, and swimming.

Extended stay trips are those where you might want to spend at least one night. Bear in mind, though, that some or all of the attractions at any of these places can be enjoyed as a daytrip as well.

Year-round spot designates a destination whose features remain appealing winter and summer alike.

Local transport refers to trolley or shuttle service sometimes provided by towns where traffic and parking can be a problem during the busy season. This service often incurs a single fee for all-day riding privileges.

One-stop attraction designates a location where you can park your car and walk to all the nearby attractions.

Nonwalking tours employ buses, trains, and boats to tour cities, towns, and harbors.

Off-season specials apply to areas where discounts are especially good and where area tourist merchants participate in special off-season activities, such as Christmas festivals.

Handicapped accessibility is indicated for those locations that advertise themselves as having facilities for the physically impaired. Locations not having this designation in the chart still offer some degree of handicapped accessibility. Attractions with many stairs or other difficult terrain are so described in the chapters.

TRIPS AT A GLANCE

	\<br\>*Antiques/auctions*	ATTRACTIONS \<br\>*Classes/workshops*	\<br\>*Crafts*	\<br\>*Gardens/farms*	\<br\>*Hiking*	\<br\>*Historic sites*	\<br\>*Museums*	\<br\>*"Old-fashioned" fun*	\<br\>*Park/nature area*	\<br\>*Performing arts*	\<br\>*Scenic area*	\<br\>*Shopping (misc.)*	\<br\>*Water sports*	PLANNING AIDS \<br\>*Daytrip*	\<br\>*Extended stay*	\<br\>*Year-round spot*	\<br\>*Local transport*	\<br\>*One-stop attraction*	\<br\>*Guided tours*	\<br\>*Nonwalking tours*	\<br\>*Handicap access*	\<br\>*Off-season specials*	\<br\>*Senior discounts*
CONNECTICUT																							
Fairfield/Westport, p. 15		●	●		●				●	●			●	●	●	●							●
Northeast Corner, p. 21	●			●		●			●		●			●		●			●				●
Route 7, p. 28		●	●				●			●	●	●	●	●	●	●							
RHODE ISLAND																							
Narragansett, p. 34			●			●					●	●	●	●					●	●		●	
MASSACHUSETTS																							
Sandwich, p. 40		●		●	●	●	●	●	●					●	●				●		●		●
Boston, p. 47						●	●			●				●	●	●	●	●	●	●	●		
Salem, p. 54						●	●					●		●	●	●	●	●	●	●	●	●	●
Rockport, p. 63		●			●		●		●	●	●	●				●	●		●			●	
Sheffield, p. 71	●		●		●	●		●	●		●		●	●		●			●				
Williamstown/N. Adams, p. 76		●			●		●			●	●			●	●	●			●	●		●	
NEW HAMPSHIRE																							
Canterbury, p. 84		●	●	●		●	●				●			●					●	●			
Meredith, p. 88	●						●			●	●	●	●	●						●			●
Franconia Notch, p. 94				●		●			●		●			●	●	●						●	●
Franconia/Sugar Hill, p. 100					●	●				●	●			●	●	●						●	●
Hanover, p. 106		●	●			●	●			●	●			●	●	●		●	●				
VERMONT																							
Route 30, p. 112	●			●	●		●	●	●		●			●	●				●				
Windsor, p. 119	●	●	●	●	●	●				●	●			●					●		●		
Weston, p. 124		●	●		●		●			●			●	●	●	●			●		●		
Middlebury, p. 131		●	●	●			●	●		●	●	●		●	●	●			●				●
Shelburne, p. 137			●	●		●	●	●	●					●		●				●	●	●	
Burlington, p. 144							●			●				●						●	●		●
MAINE																							
Freeport, p. 150		●	●					●			●	●	●	●	●								
Bath, p. 156		●	●			●			●					●		●	●			●			●
Castine, p. 161		●	●		●	●	●			●	●		●		●			●	●	●			
Blue Hill, p. 167		●	●	●						●	●	●		●	●								

PLANNING YOUR TRAVELS / 13

CONNECTICUT

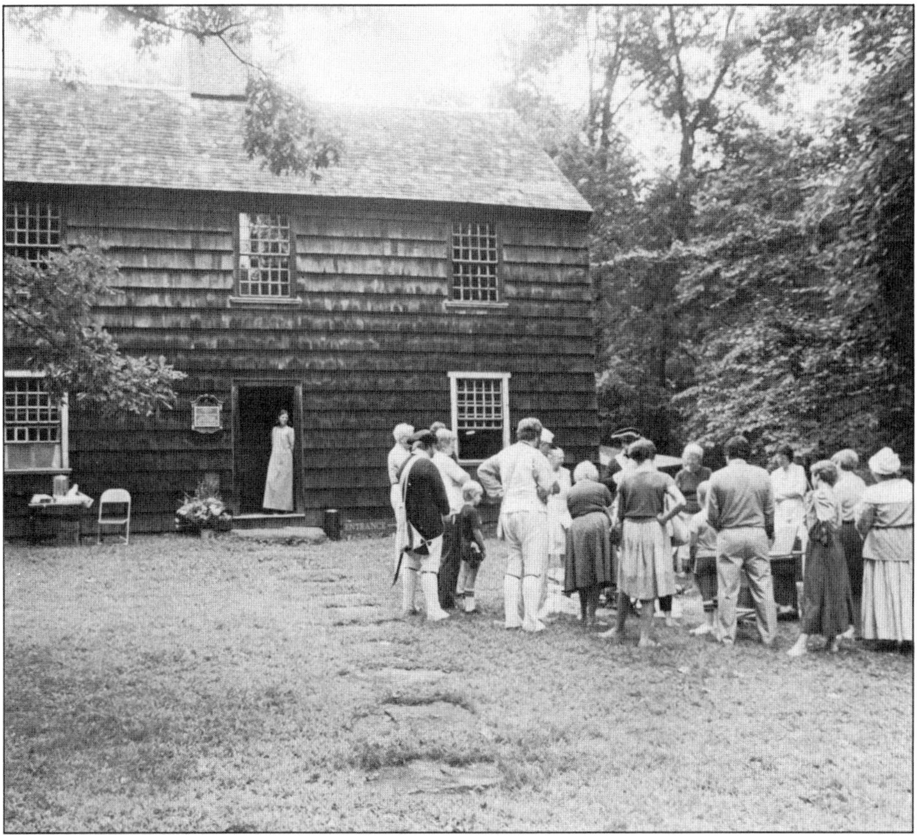

Demonstrations of eighteenth-century crafts, given at the Fairfield Historical Society's Ogden House as part of the annual August Colonial Craft Day, always draw a crowd.

Fairfield and Westport

Fairfield and Westport, both within commuting distance of Manhattan, are home to many business people who work in the Big Apple. Fairfield, burned flat by British troops in 1779 following its refusal to submit to royal authority, is a good place to explore a slice of Connecticut history. Affluent, fashionable Westport is characterized by elegant stores and lovely residential neighborhoods. Taken together, they provide a sampling of New England's southern corner — sophisticated and congested, yet endowed with attractive open spaces and good access to the pleasures of Long Island Sound. Discover

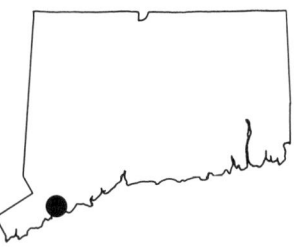

CONNECTICUT / 15

Discover them at your own pace, varying visits to historic buildings with time out to walk in the woods or relax at the shore.

them at your own pace, varying visits to historic buildings with time out to walk in the woods or relax at the shore.

In Fairfield, you can learn about early American domestic life at the **Ogden House.** This austere saltbox was built in 1750 on family land for David Ogden, who moved into it with his wife, Jane, that spring. Together they worked hard, producing most of the food and textiles required to feed and clothe their seven children. They were rewarded with a moderately prosperous lifestyle that allowed them to sip imported wines on special occasions. Although their home seems simple, keep in mind that in the eighteenth century few families owned window curtains, pewter, and substantial quantities of linens.

Ogden House is particularly intriguing to visit because it is furnished in accordance with an inventory of household possessions compiled in 1775 when David Ogden died at age forty-eight. According to the inventory, the family owned, among other items, a silver-hilted sword and a tin candle box, and such objects are now on display in the house. Many of the pieces in the collection, including a Queen Anne cherry desk and high chest, were owned by early Fairfield residents. Your costumed guide will explain that each room was used for several purposes, with family members often moving furniture from one place to another — window to fireplace, for example — depending on their needs for light, warmth, and work or recreation space. In the lean-to kitchen, you'll get a sense of how Jane Ogden spent much of her time, making cheese, baking bread, salting pork, and otherwise preparing and preserving foods.

Designed in the English style with symmetrical layout and raised beds, the re-created eighteenth-century garden is planted with small vegetables and more than forty types of herbs. Perennials and annuals, herbs were used for medicinal and culinary purposes, as insect repellent, and for dyeing fabrics. All the plants in the garden are appropriate to the period, but the collection is more varied than that found typically in a colonial garden. Take a few minutes to cross the bridge that spans the brook and to walk the wildflower trail.

It's particularly rewarding to visit the house on the annual **Colonial Craft Day,** held on a Sunday in early August, when about thirty area craftspeople demonstrate their skills and offer their work for sale on the shaded grounds surrounding the house. Many of the crafts represent tasks that were a regular part of eighteenth-century farm life. Some of the techniques demonstrated in recent years are wood-carving, quilting, rug hooking, broom making, wheat weaving, beekeeping, and smocking. Perhaps you'll have a chance to snack on homemade gingerbread and lemonade while watching the 5th Connecticut Regiment, dressed in authentic revolutionary war garb, execute drills, and while listening to the eighteenth-century military music performed by a fife and drum corps.

Another yearly Fairfield event is the **Annual Dogwood Festival,** sponsored by the Ladies Guild of the Greenfield Hill Congregational Church. The week-long festival is held in early May when the dogwood trees are in bloom. It offers a walking tour of several gardens near the church, in addition to an art show, a sit-down luncheon, and booths selling handmade items and home-baked goods. Write or call the Fairfield Chamber of Commerce for exact dates.

In addition to overseeing Ogden House, the **Fairfield Historical Society** operates its own museum, where it displays items of historic and artistic interest that pertain to the town of Fairfield and its environs, from its founding in 1639 to the present. "Gardens of the Golden Age" is typical of the society's rotating exhibits. Using old photographs, the show documents the influx of wealthy city dwellers into mid-nineteenth-century Fairfield. These affluent newcomers favored the naturalistic style of landscape design then in vogue. They built Gothic, Italianate, and Grecian style cottages and villas and hired landscape architects to design accompanying gardens and walkways and clumps of shade trees. Grandeur and sublimity were buzzwords of the day.

The back gallery includes an eclectic selection of furnishings and accessories, varying from a graceful high chest of drawers attributed to eighteenth-century Fairfield cabinetmaker Justin Hobart, Sr., to early cradles and grandfather clocks. There is also a collection of walking sticks from all over the world: an 1893 Chicago World's Fair twisted amber glass number that looks like a serpent; a birch stick with a wooden head that looks like a cigar store Indian; and a stick with a carved alligator for a handle. Still others are made of briarroot, coffee-bush wood, Cape buffalo horn, and bamboo.

If you would like to take a self-guided walking tour encompassing some of Fairfield's historic buildings, ask for a free leaflet in the museum library. Points of interest include **St. Paul's Church,** built in

Snack on homemade gingerbread and lemonade while watching the 5th Connecticut Regiment, dressed in authentic revolutionary war garb, execute drills.

The Audubon Society's 152-acre wildlife sanctuary offers six miles of hiking trails.

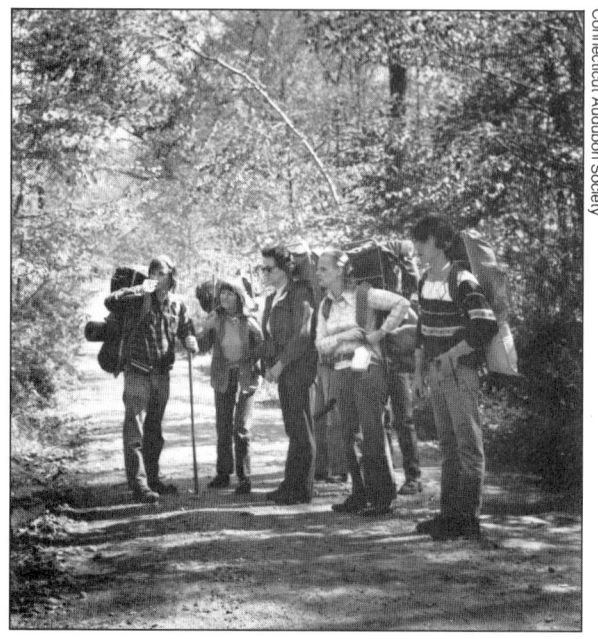

1856 on the foundation of the first town jail; the **Sun Tavern,** which entertained George Washington on his way to Boston; and the **Burr Mansion,** built in 1790 to replace the original house on the site, which was burned by the British and in which Dorothy Quincy married John Hancock, president of the Continental Congress.

For a glimpse of the local countryside, take a fifteen-minute drive out to the **Connecticut Audubon Society Fairfield Center,** a 152-acre wildlife sanctuary with six miles of trails to hike. Begin at the nature store gift shop, where you can purchase a guide to the sanctuary. The shop also stocks bird feeders, binoculars, decoys, and garden statuary, along with playing cards, note paper, mailboxes, welcome mats, coasters, clocks, napkins, and much more, all decorated with the bird motif.

The booklet describes the habitats found at nine selected stops along the trails, which wind through fields and woodlands, passing by ponds, streams, and marshes and over rocky outcrops. The Audubon Society has considerately placed numbered benches at each of these locations so that you will know you're in the right place and can rest a bit while you read the related information. The booklet gives you a choice of three routes: a thirty-minute loop, an hour loop, and a two-and-a-half-hour trip to the farther reaches of the sanctuary.

Connecticut Audubon also operates the **Birdcraft Museum and Sanctuary**, several miles away. Established as a sanctuary in 1914, this was the first private songbird refuge in New England. Exhibits include life-size dioramas showing birds and animals in their natural habitats, as well as an African room featuring stuffed antelope, rhinoceros, and lion heads. There is also a short-loop trail to walk.

In neighboring Westport, **Sherwood Island State Park** sports a mile and a half of sandy beach overlooking the sound. When you enter the park, you have a choice between East Beach and West Beach parking areas. West Beach is smaller and less attractive, and organized groups that arrive by bus are required to park at this end of the park, so it tends to get crowded. But it does have picnic tables set beneath shade trees. Here you'll also find the pavilion, which contains a snack bar; a small store selling grills, suntan lotion, and the like; and tables and chairs where you can eat out of the sun.

East Beach is nearly treeless, an expansive stretch of beach with plenty of room to spread out. The sand slopes gradually toward the shoreline, offering easy access to the water. Here you'll find men's and women's dressing rooms and another snack bar, along with an all-important sign that records the tides and air and water temperatures.

Shopping is a popular Westport activity, and you'll make your own discoveries as you stroll along streets lined with elegant shops. One store, however, is particularly worth mentioning, partly because of its very special nature and partly because its location doesn't make it a likely discovery. The **Save the Children Craft Shop** is one arm of Save the Children, the nonprofit organization that finds sponsors for children in need throughout much of the world. The shop provides a market for goods produced in self-help, community-based programs in countries where Save the Children works. In Pakistan, for example, the Craft Export Program helps Afghan women in refugee camps to earn an income by providing them with professional design and marketing guidance to make crafts suitable for export. Many of these women are skilled in traditional Afghan spinning and needlework techniques, and through this project they learn to adapt their crafts to the American market, as evidenced by the pillow covers and area rugs sold in the shop.

Visiting the shop is like visiting an international street bazaar. Colorful displays of sculpture, handwoven clothing, shiny copper bowls and bells, and

Visiting the Save the Children Craft Shop is like visiting an international street bazaar.

all sorts of baskets, toys, and pottery sit, hang, and are piled in every available space. There are hand-painted wooden musicians from Mexico, an oval mirror with a lacquered frame painted with tiny animals from Kashmir, a ceremonial jar from Nigeria, handwoven silk scarves from Sri Lanka, and carved salad servers with giraffe and elephant handles from Kenya. Our favorite piece was a wall hanging from Colombia, a seaside scene with three-dimensional stuffed swimmers attached to the beach and the artist's name signed in embroidery — one-of-a-kind folk art for certain. When you make a purchase at the Save the Children shop, you take home something wonderful and at the same time feel as though you're doing something good for the world. Altogether a satisfying experience!

Come evening, head for the **Westport Country Playhouse** in downtown Westport. A tradition spanning more than three decades, the theater produces a series of comedies and musicals throughout the summer, featuring professional actors, many of them familiar faces from both television and movie screens. The theater seats 798, with 554 seats in the orchestra and the rest upstairs. Audience members sit on long red benches (with backs) and in bentwood chairs in the upstairs boxes. Attending a performance is a festive event, as people gather in the courtyard before the show to snack on ice cream or sip a cool drink on a warm summer evening.

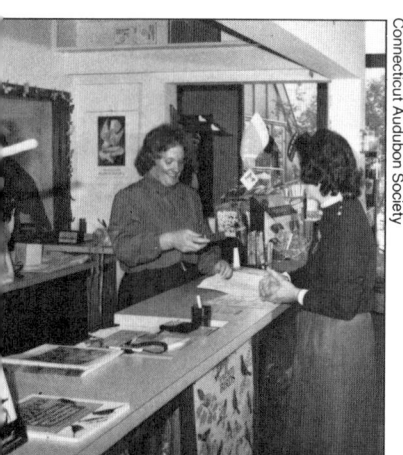

For gift items and novelties with a bird motif — from playing cards to welcome mats to napkins — stop by the Audubon Society's nature store.

ACCESS

FAIRFIELD. Take I-95 to exit 22.

WESTPORT. Take I-95 to exit 18. Follow signs to Westport.

OGDEN HOUSE. Directions: Take I-95 to exit 20. Turn right onto Bronson Road. House is located at 1520 Bronson Road. **Season:** Mid-May through mid-October. **Admission:** Charged; senior discount. **Telephone:** (203) 259-1598.

FAIRFIELD HISTORICAL SOCIETY. Directions: Follow I-95 to exit 22. Follow Route 1 (Post Road) north to intersection with Old Post Road. Turn right onto Old Post Road. Museum is located at 636 Old Post Road. **Season:** Year-round. **Admission:** Charged; senior discount. **Telephone:** (203) 259-1598.

CONNECTICUT AUDUBON SOCIETY FAIRFIELD CENTER. Directions: Follow I-95 to exit 21. Travel north on Mill Plain Road, which becomes Burr Street. Sanctuary is located at 2325 Burr Street, about 4 miles from I-95. **Season:** Year-round; closed Mondays. **Admission:** Charged. **Telephone:** (203) 259-6305.

CONNECTICUT AUDUBON SOCIETY BIRDCRAFT MUSEUM AND SANCTUARY. Directions: Follow I-95 to exit 21. Follow Mill Plain Road north. Turn right on Unquowa Road. Center is at 314 Unquowa Road. **Season:** Year-round; limited hours. **Admission:** Charged. **Telephone:** (203) 259-0416.

SHERWOOD ISLAND STATE PARK. Directions: Follow I-95 to exit 18. Follow signs to park. **Season:** Year-round. **Admission:** Charged. **Telephone:** (203) 226-6983.

SAVE THE CHILDREN CRAFT SHOP. Directions: Follow Route 1 (Post Road East) north through the center of Westport. Turn right on Route 33 just after crossing the Saugatuck River. The store is almost immediately on your right. **Season:** Year-round. **Admission:** Free. **Telephone:** (203) 226-7271.

WESTPORT COUNTRY PLAYHOUSE. Directions: Located on Route 1 (Post Road East) in Westport. **Season:** June through September. **Admission:** Charged. **Telephone:** (203) 227-5137.

For further information or restaurant and lodging suggestions, contact the Westport Chamber of Commerce, 15 Imperial Avenue, P.O. Box 30, Westport, CT 06881, (203) 227-9234; or the Fairfield Chamber of Commerce, 1597 Post Road, Fairfield, CT 06430, (203) 255-1011.

The Northeast Corner

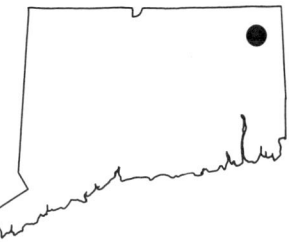

Spend a relaxed day in the countryside discovering the tucked-away pleasures of Connecticut's often overlooked northeast corner. Only a one-and-a-half-hour drive from Boston and less than an hour from Providence and Hartford, the tiny towns of Woodstock and Pomfret, characterized by corn fields, cow pastures, roadside stands, and graceful colonial buildings, feel much farther removed from the fast-paced hustle and bustle of urban life. Though serene and unhurried, this area is not without its surprises. For example, you'll find opportunities to learn the ins and outs of viniculture and wine making, as well as the fine points of African violet cultivation. Well suited for a late spring or an autumn visit, this quiet corner is also a good getaway on a perfect summer day when many other areas are unpleasantly overcrowded.

The main attraction in rural Woodstock, **Bowen House,** also known as **Roseland Cottage,** is almost impossible to miss because of its bright pink color. The house has always been painted a shade on the purple-to-rose spectrum, sometimes a muddy shade

Only a one-and-a-half-hour drive from Boston, the tiny towns of Woodstock and Pomfret feel much farther removed from the hustle and bustle of urban life.

of pink, sometimes a bright, bubble-gum pink. Called Roseland Cottage because of both its color and the roses cultivated in its garden, the house was built by Henry C. Bowen, born in Woodstock in 1813, whose father kept the local country store and post office. At age twenty-one, Henry set off for New York City to seek his fortune — with great success, as it turned out. He became an affluent businessman and later directed his energies toward *The Independent*, a Congregationalist weekly that he helped found. In addition to Congregationalism, he believed in abolition, patriotism, and the Republican party.

Bowen commissioned English-born architect Joseph Collins Wells to design a summer residence for him in his hometown. Wells was primarily known for his Gothic style church designs, an interest reflected in Roseland Cottage's ornamental woodwork in forms such as pointed arches, trefoil and quatrefoil motifs, and the brightly colored stained-glass windows. Wells even designed the fancy fence along the roadway in the Gothic style.

The 1846 house sits on its original two-and-a-half-acre plot, across from Woodstock Common, where Bowen's sons played polo. The rest of the family favored croquet on the lawn, enjoying proximity to the parterre garden, which has twenty-one flower beds. The garden is edged with a boxwood hedge that descends back to the original six hundred yards of hedge planted in 1850. The Society for the Preservation of New England Antiquities, which owns and manages Roseland Cottage, plants some four thousand annuals each year, basing their placement on Bowen's original plans. Your visit to the house itself takes the form of a forty-minute guided tour. Several steps lead into the house, and you'll have to climb a full flight of stairs to reach the bedrooms. All the furniture in the house was used by the family at one time or another, and the pieces in the first parlor were designed by the architect. All the windows in the two parlors — much of the glass bright red, purple, green, blue, yellow, or orange — could be opened from top and bottom so air could circulate freely in hot weather. In the conservatory you'll see one of the lanterns Bowen used to illuminate the grounds on the Fourth of July, when he particularly enjoyed expressing his patriotic spirit.

Roseland Cottage was often filled with people. You'll see a portrait of Bowen's first wife, Lucy, who died of complications following the birth of their tenth child. Bowen remarried and had another child.

Henry Bowen's Roseland Cottage, built in 1813, takes its name from the surrounding rose gardens and from the building's eye-catching pink exterior.

Between Bowen's own huge brood and visiting relatives, Roseland was alive with activity. In addition, Bowen liked to entertain. His guests included four United States presidents, Ulysses S. Grant, Rutherford B. Hayes, Benjamin Harrison, and William McKinley, all of whom attended his famous Fourth of July celebrations.

Continuing to tour the house, you'll discover that many of the walls are covered with Lincrusta Walton, a wallpaper technique invented by Frederick Walton, who also invented linoleum. Meant to look like tooled leather work, the paper has a raised or embossed effect. Pictures of cherubs adorn the wall in the master bedroom, and the faces are those of Bowen's grandchildren. Now it's on to the dining room, where the table is set with red-and-white Limoges china made especially for this house, with Henry Bowen's initials in the center of nearly every piece. Limoges serving dishes sit on the ornate rococo sideboard.

On your way upstairs, you'll pass several important-looking framed documents on the hallway wall. One is a letter signed by Abraham Lincoln appointing Henry Bowen tax collector for the district. Upstairs you'll view several more bedrooms, two of them furnished with simple cottage furniture, some of it painted to look like carved Gothic pieces. The "Presidents' Bedroom," where the presidents were put up when they came to visit, has an unusually complete set of chamberware, including slop bucket, chamber pot, shaving mug, basins, bowl, and soap dish. It also has a lovely view of the garden.

House tour completed, head for the outbuildings. There's an elegant icehouse and privy, but the

> *The crown jewel is the wooden bowling alley, the earliest private alley in the United States still in existence.*

crown jewel is the wooden bowling alley, the earliest private alley in the United States still in existence. The pins are wood, and along the wall sit wooden balls of many sizes. As the story goes, President Grant bowled here. Briefly. Seems he rolled one ball, a strike no less. Then he decided he needed a cigarette. Henry Bowen would have none of that, however, and he sent his guest outside to smoke. Grant was so annoyed he refused to continue the game.

Less than a mile from Roseland Cottage, **Fox Hunt Farms** sells farm-fresh produce, imported cheeses, crusty French bread, and fresh fudge made right on the spot. They'll happily put up a picnic for you to take along on your travels. A good place to enjoy your picnic is **Roseland Park,** constructed by Henry Bowen in 1876 as a gift to Woodstock residents and in honor of the one hundredth anniversary of the signing of the Declaration of Independence. Located about a mile and a half from Roseland Cottage, the park has several wooden tables near the edge of an attractive pond.

If you are intrigued by African violets, you'll want to make a brief sidetrip (fifteen-minute drive) to **Buell's Greenhouses** in Eastford, where more than eight hundred kinds of African violets flourish in a complex of seven greenhouses encompassing half an acre of growing space. Here you'll find all sorts of exotic and rare varieties, from miniature to full size. It's hard to imagine there could be so many shades of pink, purple, and blue. The plants, 160,000 strong, seem to bloom everywhere, from tiny pots to hanging baskets. There are also related varieties: hybrid gloxinias, achimenes, columneas, episcias, miniature sinningias, terrarium plants, and more. No

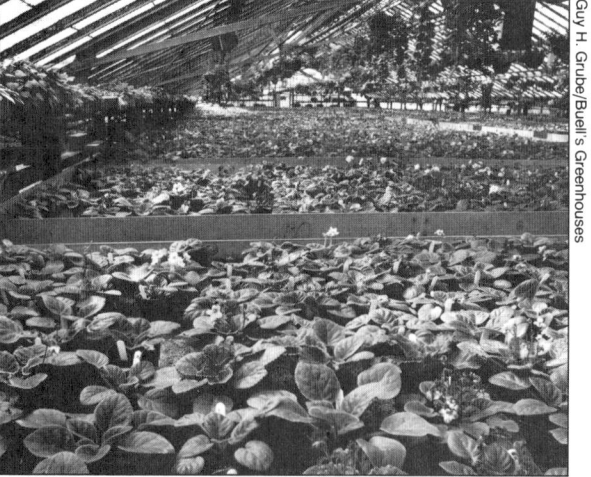

More than eight hundred varieties of African violets flourish at Buell's Greenhouses in Eastford.

24 / CONNECTICUT

matter how large your African violet collection, you're sure to find some unusual additions.

Related books and horticulture supplies are sold as well. Whether you've cultivated African violets and their relatives for years or are just starting, this is the place to stock up on both plants and advice. You'll find out all you need to know about providing adequate light, water, humidity, and food. Ask too about how to propagate your plants through leaf cuttings and offset sprouts. If you've had problems with pests, diseases, or crown rot, this is the place to turn for help.

Now it's time to take a short drive through farm country to nearby Pomfret. Don't worry if the weather is less than perfect; there's nothing quite so cozy on a rainy day as poking through a stuffed-to-the-gills attic. That's what it's like visiting **Pomfret Antique World**, where you'll unearth all sorts of treasures, from the utilitarian to the purely fanciful to the "what's this?" Fifty antique dealers share space under one roof here, and the merchandise offered is as diverse as their tastes and interests. Antique furniture shares space with small collectibles, including items to fit budgets slim and padded.

Hamlet Hill Vineyards, just yards away from Pomfret Antique World, knows how to treat visitors. This is one winery where you'll really feel welcome. Begin by watching a twelve-minute introductory video in the round theater, where the walls are covered with paper patterned in wine labels. Produced on the grounds at Hamlet Hill and at the vineyards three miles away, much of the film is narrated by the resident wine maker. You'll learn that fifteen kinds of grapes are grown here and that six tons of grapes are crushed in a single hour. Since fermentation begins within twenty-four hours of crushing, the young wines have to be monitored very closely, undergoing nearly constant analysis in the lab. But no matter how sophisticated the testing and lab work, when it comes to selecting just the right moment for bottling, the wine maker must rely on his own senses of sight, smell, and taste. The film provides close-ups of every phase of wine making, including footage of the harvest and the crushing and bottling processes.

When the film is over, take a walk around the semicircular wooden deck that overlooks the winemaking area. The activity you see depends on the time of day and the particular production schedule. Clearly labeled signs explain that this is a family winery, meaning that while some of the grapes are

Take a walk inside the immense hundred-year-old wooden wine cask, then try your skill with the hand-corker.

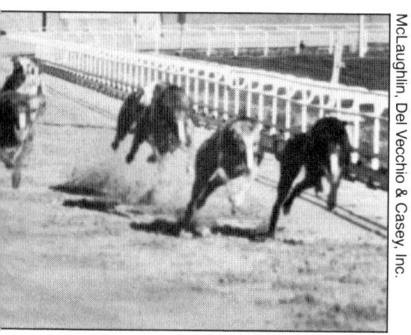

Not even the swiftest thoroughbreds could keep pace with these sleek speedsters at Plainfield Greyhound Park.

McLaughlin, Del Vecchio & Casey, Inc.

purchased from other Connecticut growers, most come from the owner's own vineyards, just up the road. The soil in this area was made by glaciers fifty thousand years ago, and glacial till makes one of the best environments for growing fine wine grapes.

Another panel explains that the grapes are picked by hand, crushed without delay, and immediately inoculated with pure natural wine yeast grown in the on-site lab by the resident chemist — the wine maker. You'll learn how temperature during fermentation affects the flavor of the wine, and you'll learn about the aging and clarification processes. If there's bottling or labeling in progress, you'll be able to get a good look by peering down one of the special observation windows aimed at this part of the cellar. Before leaving the deck, take a walk inside the immense hundred-year-old wooden wine cask, then try your skill with the hand-corker. This is the very same machine that was used to bottle all of the first year's production at Hamlet Hill.

In the retail showroom, stand at the wooden bar and sample five or six of the wines produced here. Wines are available for purchase, by the bottle or by the case, along with baskets packed with wine, wineglasses, and a corkscrew. You can bring along your own picnic lunch, or you can call the winery a day ahead and they'll have a Fox Hunt Farms lunch waiting for you when you arrive. Then pick out a bottle of wine to enjoy with your meal at one of the picnic tables down by the stream. The shop also stocks cookbooks, books about wine, titles related to plant propagation, and local food specialties such as all-natural Woodstock Preserves, which come attractively packaged in glass jars with calico-covered lids. Choose from wild blueberry jam, red currant jelly, and blackberry jam, for starters.

When you've finished tasting and shopping, take a walk in the adjacent experimental vineyard. Four varieties of grapes are grown on this quarter-acre plot, planted in 1982. The two hundred vines include Chardonnay, Riesling, White Rogue, and Verdelet, and a series of signs provides a bit of information about the history and growth requirements of each one.

Want to cap your day with a little excitement? You'll find it at the **Plainfield Greyhound Park,** where the sleek canines run up to 45 mph, outclocking even the speediest racehorses. Races, which flash by in thirty to forty seconds, take place every fifteen minutes. In between you'll have enough time to place your bet. You can wager to win, place, or show, or you can try your luck at the more sophisticated combinations involved in the daily double, trifectas, and quinellas. Watch the races from right down by the track or go to one of the restaurant facilities and watch through the viewing windows or on an individual miniscreen beside your table. Racing takes place both afternoons and evenings, with the specific schedule varying according to the time of year.

ACCESS

WOODSTOCK. Follow I-395 to Putnam/Route 44 exit. Follow Route 44 west to Route 169. Take Route 169 north into Woodstock.

POMFRET. Follow I-395 to exit 93. Take Route 101 west for 5 miles.

BOWEN HOUSE (ROSELAND COTTAGE). Directions: Located on Route 169/17, facing the Woodstock Common. **Season:** Late May through mid-September, afternoons only; mid-September to mid-October, weekends. **Admission:** Charged; senior discount. **Telephone:** (203) 928-4074.

FOX HUNT FARMS. Directions: Located on Route 169/17, across from the Woodstock Fairgrounds. **Season:** Year-round. **Admission:** Free. **Telephone:** (203) 928-0714.

ROSELAND PARK. Directions: From Roseland Cottage, follow Route 169 south to traffic island. Turn left in front of large yellow house, then immediately left again. Continue 1 mile to park on right. **Season:** Late May through mid-October. **Admission:** Free. **Telephone:** None.

BUELL'S GREENHOUSES. Directions: From the intersection of Routes 101 and 169 in Pomfret, go west on Route 101, which will become Route 44. Continue several miles to Route 198. Turn right on Route 198, then left on Westford Road. Turn right on Weeks Road to greenhouses. **Season:** Year-round. **Admission:** Free. **Telephone:** (203) 974-0623.

POMFRET ANTIQUE WORLD. Directions: Located on Route 101 in Pomfret Center. **Season:** Year-round; closed Wednesdays. **Admission:** Free. **Telephone:** (203) 928-5006.

HAMLET HILL VINEYARDS. Directions: Located on Route 101 in Pomfret, just west of the intersection with Route 169. **Season:** Year-round. **Admission:** Free. **Telephone:** (203) 928-5550.

PLAINFIELD GREYHOUND PARK. Directions: Located just off I-395 at exit 87, Plainfield. **Season:** Year-round. **Admission:** Charged. **Telephone:** (203) 564-3391.

For further information or restaurant and lodging suggestions, contact the Northeast Corner Visitors District, Box 9, Chase Road, Thompson, CT 06277. Telephone: (203) 923-2998.

Both novice and experienced craftspeople have received expert instruction for more than thirty years at the Brookfield Craft Center.

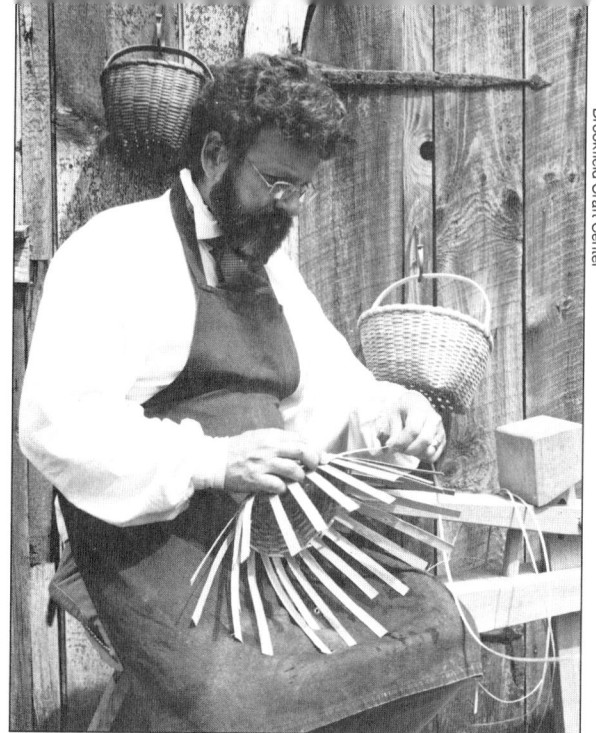

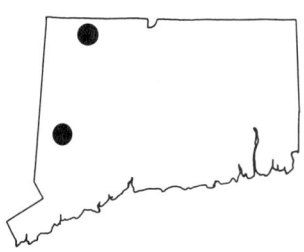

Route 7: Brookfield to Norfolk

Some vacations provide pure and simple relaxation, an opportunity to rest and feel renewed by virtue of doing very little in a lovely place. Others are physically demanding. Still another kind of vacation provides the opportunity to exercise creative talents, to learn a new skill, or to refine an old one in the company of fellow students who share the joy of learning.

Western Connecticut has two outstanding schools that offer classes suitable for vacationers. Unlike traditional courses, these classes or workshops last from one day to a week. Offered year-round, they provide an excellent getaway whenever you feel the urge to hit the road. Single travelers will find them an excellent way to meet people with similar interests. Between classes you can explore the pastoral towns and villages that line rural Route 7, which make it hard to believe you are only a few hours from New York City. Come evening, you may want to relax with some fine music.

Founded in 1954 to "preserve and promote an interest in and the learning of the skills of the American craftsman," the **Brookfield Craft Center** offers classes, workshops, seminars, exhibits, demonstrations, and other craft-related events. Located on the banks of the Still River, the Brookfield campus comprises four eighteenth- and nineteenth-century buildings, the oldest of which is a restored gristmill dating back to about 1780.

Serving both accomplished and novice craftspeople, the center has earned a reputation as one of the finest nonacademic craft education schools in the United States. More than four hundred classes and workshops are held each year, here and at the branch facility recently opened in South Norwalk. Students of all ages come from around the country and abroad to study with an impressive line-up of internationally acclaimed craftspeople.

Courses are offered year-round, and most of the programs last one, two, or three days. While tuition and fees vary, they generally average about fifty dollars a day. Some courses last a week or longer. A catalog listing the courses for the coming season is published quarterly. A recent edition of the catalog included programs in basketry, bird carving, boatbuilding, clay design and marketing, fabric and quilting, fiber and weaving, glass, metals and jewelry, paper, photography, special interest, and wood.

Here's a sample course description:

Bird Carving for Beginners
Sat. and Sun. 10–4.

This special weekend course has been specifically designed to make it "easy" for beginners to reach the "first plateau" of bird carving by making a decoy type bird. The only tools needed will be a hand held jigsaw and Xacto knife with #22 blades. Students will be guided step-by-step through the selection of wood, the making of patterns, the cutting of blanks, the shaping and smoothing of the form, the setting of eyes, and the final painting and finishing. Participants should be able to complete an antiqued Blue Billed Decoy during this weekend.

Even if you are not ready to sign up for a course, stop by the Brookfield Craft Center to visit the shop and see the current exhibit in the gallery, which features work by some of the finest craftspeople in the country, be they bladesmiths (knife makers), enamelists, woodturners, or photographers. The shop is filled with intriguing handcrafted objects such as leaded-glass boxes, ceramic mobiles, wrought-iron fireplace tools, handwoven eyeglass cases, painted wooden mirror frames, brass jewelry, and hand-

Even if you are not ready to sign up for a course, stop by the Brookfield Craft Center to visit the shop, which features work by some of the finest craftspeople in the country.

printed scarves. From Thanksgiving to Christmas Eve, the shop is markedly enlarged, with several thousand finely crafted items displayed on the three floors of the mill building.

If you love to cook, you'll love **The Silo** in New Milford. A down-at-the-heels farm as recently as 1972, The Silo now pulses with activity. The spruced-up stables and barns (including two towering silos) are stocked to the rafters with barbecue and picnic equipment, table linens, fine utensils, cookware, and gourmet gadgets, many items imported from Europe. Whether you fancy an iron griddle or a clay cooker, an electric brunch pan or a set of cannoli forms, The Silo has what you need. One of the silos is filled with hand-painted Portuguese pottery in soft shades of blue and brown. Elsewhere in the barn is a section stocked with specialty foods made by small businesses throughout New England. Another building contains an attractive art gallery, which features changing exhibits in varied media.

While shopping is excuse enough to visit The Silo, there is an even better reason. Here you can enroll in a seminar or workshop at The Cooking School, where classes are taught by professional chefs, cookbook authors, and restaurateurs. Some of the instructors are on the staff of the Culinary Institute of America, where they teach other chefs their profession. Most of the seminars and workshops are single-session offerings lasting three to four hours. They are scheduled on weekend evenings and afternoons year-round, providing an excellent escape from the winter doldrums or spring cabin fever.

A broad variety of culinary topics is covered.

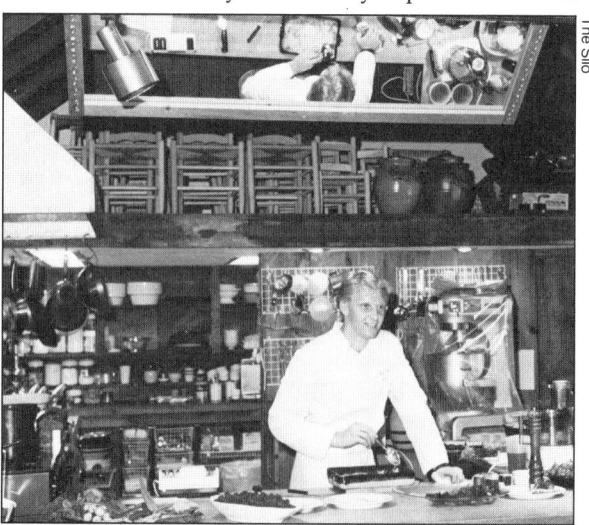

Professional chefs, cookbook authors, and restaurateurs share their expertise with students at The Silo Cooking School in New Milford.

Here are some sample course titles (to whet your appetite): "Cooking with Jacques Pepin" (Steamed Scallops in Garlic Escarole, Chicken Stuffed Under the Skin, Purée of White Beans, Raspberry Soufflé); "Madeleine Cooks at The Silo" (Madeleine Kamman prepares Jalapeño Pasta with Creamed Corn and Red Onion Sauce, Roast Veal Loin in Crumb Coat, Parmigiano Sauce with Endives, Spaghetti de Legumes, Biscuit Glacé Hawaiian Style); "Cooking That's Good for You" (a member of the U.S. Culinary Olympic Team shares recipes and techniques which prove "that excellent cuisine and healthful food can be one and the same").

Some of the courses are demonstrations, while others provide an opportunity for participation. Sampling the fare is always a popular part of the program. If you would like to enroll, write for a course listing, which includes both a general description and the actual menu for each program offered. Advance registration is strongly advised.

Between classes, there's plenty else to do in this lovely corner of Connecticut. Take a ride north along Route 7, which follows the course of the Housatonic River, and explore the villages along the way. The countryside is pleasing any time of year, but it becomes downright spectacular during foliage season in late September and October. Just south of Kent, you'll come to the **Housatonic Trading Co./Country Things,** a riverside shop overflowing with elegant and endearing pieces of folk art contributed by more than two hundred New England craftspeople. There are quilts, blankets and rugs, boxes, baskets, pottery, and toys, representing a multitude of styles. In Kent proper, Route 7 passes **Kent Station Square,** a cluster of upscale shops housed in and around a century-old railroad station. Businesses include a fine arts gallery, a classy antique shop, a pizza garden, and several boutiques. Give yourself an energy boost at **Stosh's Ice Cream,** where sampling is encouraged. Flavors like chocolate-chocolate (a not too distant cousin of chocolate mousse), lemon, and peanut butter–chocolate kiss help explain why Stosh's cool confection was recently applauded in a national publication called *The Very Best Ice Cream.*

Soon after passing through Kent, you'll come to **The Sloane-Stanley Museum,** where all the exhibits were designed by noted Connecticut artist and writer Eric Sloane, who also donated a fine collection of early tools. Sloane considered tools extensions of human hands and works of art. This attitude is reflected in the way he chose to display the collection.

Whether you fancy an iron griddle or a clay cooker, an electric brunch pan or a set of cannoli forms, The Silo has what you need.

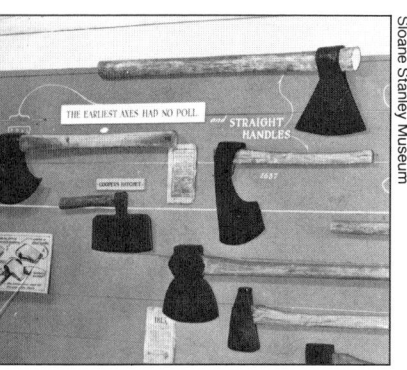

Eric Sloane donated and chose the display setting for the hand tools on exhibit at the Sloane-Stanley museum in Kent.

Displayed on bare wooden platforms against a background of barn boards painted subdued blue, tan, or barn red, the wooden corset stays, oaken scrub board, and birch broom command the same respect as sculpture in an art museum.

Be sure to stop in at the adjacent cabin on the property, which represents the home of Noah, the subject of Sloane's beloved book, *Diary of an Early American Boy*. The book is based on a small wood-backed, leather-bound diary that Sloane found, and the cabin, with its dirt floor and simple furnishings (the ladder leading up to the loft is carved from a tree trunk), gives a feeling for how Noah lived.

Continuing north on Route 7, you'll come to **Kent Falls State Park,** where the big attraction is the two-hundred-foot cascade of sparkling water that plunges into the stream by the grassy picnic area. A steep trail leads to the top of the falls, but you don't have to climb it to enjoy the sight and sound of rushing water. Picnicking, fishing, and hiking are the main activities.

At **Music Mountain** in Falls Village you can hear wonderful music that varies from Gilbert and Sullivan to folk to chamber music. Recent performers have included the Westport Madrigal Singers, the Little City String Band, the American Music/Theatre Group, and one of the Soviet Union's leading string quartets.

If you would like to assemble a preconcert picnic, head for **Harris Foods, Ltd.,** in nearby Salisbury. Their "gourmet to go" division will happily put up a scrumptious lunch or dinner. Choose from sandwiches, quiches, soups, salads, fine cheeses, pâtés, smoked meats, and much more. And don't forget the dessert.

If you visit this part of Connecticut during the summer, you can treat yourself to a concert in a charming country setting. The **Norfolk Chamber Music Festival,** a tradition since 1941, makes its home at the Ellen Battell Stoeckel Estate in Norfolk. Some of the world's most renowned musicians, including the Tokyo String Quartet, the New York Woodwind Quintet, and the New York Brass Quintet, perform in the acoustically superb Music Shed. Audience members are invited to bring along a picnic to enjoy on the elegant grounds, where musicians often treat them to a preconcert performance. Young musicians from the Yale Summer School of Music, which runs concurrently with the festival, often perform recitals, which are free of charge. There is also an art gallery to visit.

ACCESS

BROOKFIELD CRAFT CENTER. Directions: Follow Route 7 north to Brookfield. Turn right on Route 25. The sales gallery and office are located almost immediately on your right. **Season:** Year-round. **Admission:** Free. **Telephone:** (203) 775-4526.

THE SILO. Directions: Follow Route 7 to Upland Road in New Milford. The Silo is ¼ mile east of Route 7. **Season:** Year-round. **Admission:** Free. **Telephone:** (203) 355-0300.

HOUSATONIC TRADING CO./COUNTRY THINGS. Directions: Located on Route 7 one mile south of Kent center. **Season:** Year-round. **Admission:** Free. **Telephone:** (203) 927-4411.

STOSH'S ICE CREAM. Directions: Located at Kent Station, Route 7, in Kent. **Season:** Year-round. **Admission:** Free. **Telephone:** (203) 927-4495.

THE SLOANE–STANLEY MUSEUM. Directions: Located on Route 7 just north of the center of Kent. **Season:** Mid-May through October. **Admission:** Charged; senior discount. **Telephone:** (203) 927-3628.

KENT FALLS STATE PARK. Directions: Located on Route 7, north of Kent. **Season:** Year-round. **Admission:** Free. **Telephone:** None.

MUSIC MOUNTAIN. Directions: Follow Route 7 to Route 126. Go east on Route 126 to Route 63. Follow signs to Music Mountain. **Season:** Mid-June through mid-September. **Admission:** Charged. **Telephone:** (203) 496-1222.

HARRIS FOODS, LTD. Directions: Follow Route 7 to Route 44 west, then turn left onto Academy Street. Located on Academy Street, just off Route 44, in Salisbury. **Season:** Year-round; closed February and March. **Admission:** Free. **Telephone:** (203) 435-2062.

NORFOLK CHAMBER MUSIC FESTIVAL. Directions: Follow Route 7 north to Canaan. Turn right on Route 44 and continue east to Ellen Battell Stoeckel Estate in Norfolk. **Season:** Early July through early August. **Admission:** Charged (except for some recitals). **Telephone:** (203) 432-1966 (until June 15); (203) 542-5537 (after June 15).

For further information or restaurant and lodging suggestions, contact the New Milford Chamber of Commerce, 30 Bridge Street, New Milford, CT 06776, (203) 354-6080; or the Chamber of Commerce of Northwest Connecticut, Inc., P.O. Box 59, 12 Mason Street, Torrington, CT 06790, (203) 482-6586. For information on bed and breakfast establishments in the northwest corner of Connecticut, contact Covered Bridge Bed & Breakfast, West Cornwall, CT 06796. Telephone: (203) 542-5944.

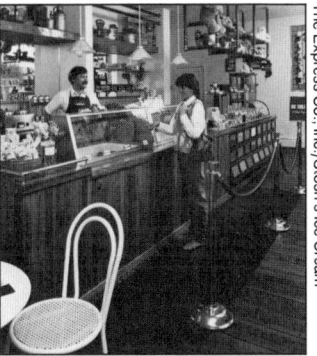

"One of everything, please!" Stosh's Ice Cream recently received national recognition in The Very Best Ice Cream.

RHODE ISLAND

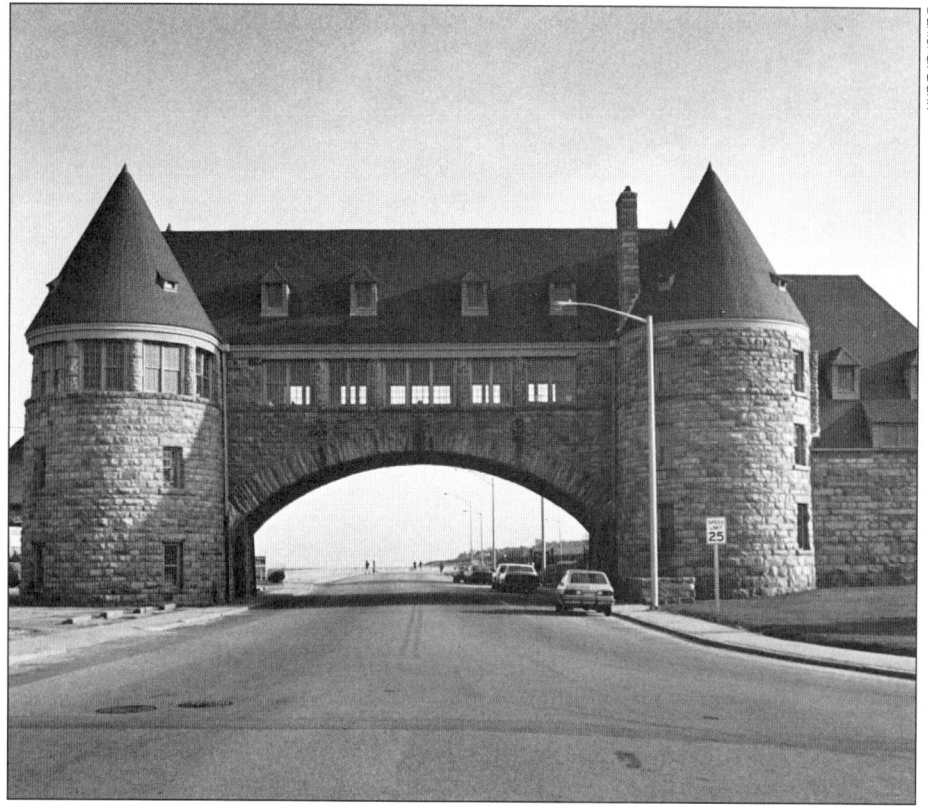

The Towers, the lone remnant of a six-story Victorian amusement complex, reminds visitors of a time when the Narragansett waterfront was a place to see and be seen.

Narragansett

Close your eyes and imagine a string of white sandy beaches, a bevy of fishing boats with hungry gulls swirling above, the freshest seafood and the saltiest air.... Welcome to Narragansett, Galilee, and Jerusalem, on the southeastern coast of Rhode Island. Crowds of vacationers flock here in July and August, but during late spring and autumn you'll find these villages relaxed and rewarding places to visit, and off-season bargain rates are in good supply.

The most prominent landmark in Narragansett is **The Towers,** a massive elevated stone promenade, anchored at each end by a conical tower, that spans Ocean Road like a bridge. Located by the edge of the water, The Towers is part of an area known as Narragansett Pier. In 1887 the *New York Times* described Narragansett Pier as "an American watering place in the truest sense of the term." Drawn by the tempting beaches, well-heeled vacationers descended on Narragansett each summer to savor the sand and surf and the manmade pleasures of the pier, most prominent of which was the Casino. More than a place to gamble, the Casino was a six-story trove of social and recreational opportunities, a place to see and be seen. It housed tennis courts, a bowling alley, billiards and card rooms, a rifle gallery, a theater and a ballroom. An orchestra played concert music during the day, and dance numbers in the evening, and there was plenty to eat and drink. The covered promenade you see stretching across the road today, connecting the two ivy-covered towers, was often filled with overflow crowds from the main dining room.

Most of the Casino complex was destroyed by fire in 1900, leaving The Towers behind as a reminder of the golden Victorian resort era. With the glamour of the past a memory, Narragansett retains its natural charm as a quiet community with lovely beaches overlooking Rhode Island Sound.

Narragansett itself has five beaches, the largest of which is **Scarborough State Beach.** Conveniences include picnic tables and a large bathhouse. The parking lots that serve this beach and the smaller ones nearby are often packed to capacity early in the day during July and August, particularly on weekends. Off-season, you won't have any problems.

Here and in surrounding South County, you'll find an abundance of accommodations: elegant inns, simple cottages, efficient motels, and intimate bed and breakfasts. The selection of restaurants is equally varied, in price, ambiance, cuisine, and setting. Stop at The Towers for advice on how to make the most of your visit and to examine a collection of menus. (If you plan to arrive at the height of the season, lodging reservations well in advance are a must.)

"The most magnificent time to visit us and our beaches is in September and October. May and June are beautiful, too," explains long-time resident Jack Gaines, who heads up the tourism board for Narragansett and South County and hangs his hat at The Towers. Considering that his job is to promote tourism, his next remark is most unexpected. "Stay away if you can between the end of school and Labor Day.

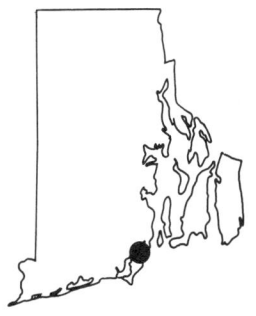

In 1887 the New York Times *described Narragansett Pier as "an American watering place in the truest sense of the term."*

"The most magnificent time to visit us and our beaches is in September and October."

We just can't handle all the visitors. Have to send some of them an hour out of town just to find them a place to sleep."

Jack Gaines is a realist. He has great affection for this area, and he values mature travelers. But he wants you to enjoy yourself, and he doesn't think that's as easy when the beaches, streets, and shops are elbow-to-elbow with visitors. As a senior citizen himself, he knows the value of a dollar and likes to get a good deal. In the summer Narragansett hotel, restaurant, and shop owners don't have to go out of their way to attract customers. People just naturally flock to the area because of its beauty, beaches, and unpretentious character. (You'll find both trendy boutiques and quaint shops selling souvenirs made from seashells, but you won't find the kind of tacky "strip" that dominates many seaside resorts.)

Come Labor Day, however, an exodus occurs. This means people in the tourist business have to try harder. Many offer specials or off-season rates. Proprietors are more relaxed, and there's time to chat with visitors without the pressure that exists in summer. So it makes good sense to follow Jack Gaines's advice. Visit pre- or post-season and take your time while stretching your vacation dollars. After all, the fish don't pack up and head south just because the kids go back to school.

The best Narragansett activity of all is wandering. Explore the shops, go to the beach, do some shore fishing, eat some absolutely fresh seafood, attend an evening concert at the gazebo in Casino Park, just steps away from The Towers. The one formal sightseeing stop you ought to leave time for is a visit to the **South County Museum,** located on Canonchet Farm. The museum chronicles the history of rural Rhode Island, focusing on early American life and industry, in the home, on the farm, and at sea.

The museum is located in a new, barnlike structure. Here you'll see the implements, utensils, tools, appliances, and mechanical devices used by craftspeople, farmers, housewives, mariners, and professional men in South County from about 1850 until about 1920. Your visit takes the form of a low-key guided tour, with plenty of opportunity to ask questions. In the general store exhibit, you'll hear that the store was the center of both social and commercial life in the town. "This was where you found out who was born, who died, who had company from out of town," your guide begins. She goes on to explain that some such stores housed a portable post office. Who got the post office concession depended on the political situation. It was transferred from one general store to another depending on whether a Republican or Democrat was in power.

In the housekeeping area you'll see helpful domestic gadgets such as a sausage stuffer, sock stretchers, a rocking butter churn, and a wooden vacuum cleaner with bellows action. The costume section displays Victorian shoes and gowns, along with some unusual stone hat forms. In the textile area, a note written by an early nineteenth-century weaver from these parts observes that "more money can be made by weaving than by farming. I have wove 30 yards of rag carpet in one day at 10 cents a yard." Other exhibits focus on boatbuilding, growing a grain crop, and several other aspects of early rural life.

The museum is located on a small working farm that belongs to the state, and you are welcome to bring a picnic to eat at one of the tables. You'll make the acquaintance of the geese, chicks, sheep, donkey, pony, and goats that live here. Then take a postlunch walk in the woods. The mile-long nature trail begins as a broad grassy track, edged by banks of thimbleberries and dense clusters of grapevines, but soon becomes a narrow, rooty path. When you come to the point where you have to make a choice, bear right. Then, almost immediately, turn left and pass through the opening in the stone wall. Follow the path a bit farther, and suddenly the woods give way to a wide open vista looking out over the salt marsh and an estuary of the Narrow River. With luck, you might sight the osprey nest.

Your history lesson completed, get back to outright recreation. Fishing is a major attraction in these parts. There are opportunities for shore surf and rock casting, as well as bottom fishing in protected bay areas. Offshore game fishing is very popular, and you won't have any difficulty finding a place on a party boat going out in search of blues, bass, cod, or flounder. If you have Ernest Hemingway delusions, you can charter a boat and launch a quest for the big stuff — tuna, shark, or marlin.

To choose a boat, take a stroll along the docks in Galilee and check out the available craft. Many have boxes of information leaflets attached to a post near where they tie up, to give you the facts even if the captain is not on hand. The chamber of commerce office in The Towers also will give you a booklet listing party and charter fishing boats so that you can call the captain ahead if you have any questions. Figure out what kind of fish you're after and how

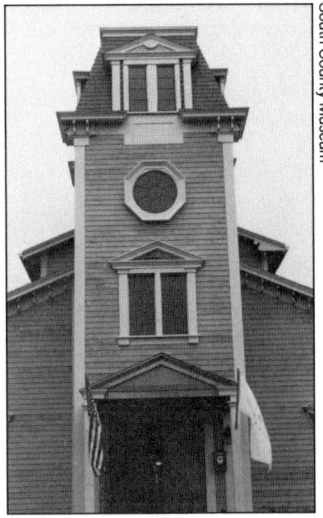

South County Museum chronicles the early American history of rural Rhode Island.

If you have Ernest Hemingway delusions, you can charter a boat and launch a quest for the big stuff — tuna, shark, or marlin.

long you want to devote to the hunt. Then sign on for a full- or half-day trip.

While you're down on the docks, you're likely to see a blackboard or two announcing current leaders in the annual **Rhode Island Party & Charter Boat Association Fishing Tournament**. As of June 30, in one recent season, some of the front-runners weighed in as follows: tautog, 14 lbs. 8 oz.; bluefish, 12 lbs. 8 oz.; mako shark, 146 lbs.

Galilee is the major departure point for ferryboats to Block Island, which means it gets very congested during the summer. Parking on the main street is difficult, and you'll probably have to use one of the pay parking lots if you visit at the height of the season. While you're in town, treat yourself to that fantastic seafood you've been dreaming about. Restaurants, snack bars, and fish markets line the main street, and the fare includes everything from full-course shore dinners to squid, snail salad, red or white chowder, jumbo shrimp, filet of sole, scrod, swordfish, clam cakes, steamers, and on and on. Many of the boats unload directly into the back doors of the markets and restaurants, so you know this seafood is just about as fresh as it gets.

In Galilee you can also climb aboard the sixty-four-foot **M/V** *Southland* for a one-and-three-quarter-hour sightseeing cruise, departing from State Pier. Cocktails and snacks are sold onboard. Viewing is best from the open upper deck, but you can also retreat to an enclosed lower deck if it gets chilly. You'll wend your way among commercial fishing boats, ferries, charter boats, and pleasure craft as your captain expounds on the social and commercial life of Jerusalem, Galilee, and Point Judith, a land mass that juts out into the ocean and is the base for a lighthouse.

When you leave Galilee, take a few minutes to detour to Jerusalem, just a few miles west. Cross Succatash Marsh and you'll see signs to **East Matunuck State Beach,** a splendid sweep of sand perfect for an afternoon of sun and salty air. Continuing into Jerusalem, you'll feel as though you've entered another world. The tiny houses line up one after another throughout the town, weather-beaten summer cottages with patches of sand and sea grass in place of lawns. Instead of gravel, broken clamshells often "pave" the paths and parking areas.

A good way to savor Jerusalem's ambiance is to have lunch at **Jim's Dockside,** a rustic yet comfortable restaurant right on the shore. Inside there's a counter with four stools and a bunch of small tables

Galilee and boats are synonymous, especially in summer when ferries depart from here on their way to popular Block Island.

covered with blue-and-white tablecloths. Or you can carry your food outside and eat on the deck directly overlooking the water. For breakfast try the massive muffins or a substantial slab of coffee cake. Later in the day, there's chowder, clam cakes, and fish sandwiches, along with hamburgers and the usual coffee shop fare. For dessert there's Pinguino's Ice Cream, made right here in Rhode Island. It comes in flavors such as apricot nectar and raspberry kir royal, and once you've tasted it, you're hooked.

ACCESS

NARRAGANSETT. Take Route 1 to Wakefield. Continue into Narragansett on Route 1A.

THE TOWERS: NARRAGANSETT INFORMATION CENTER. Directions: Located in the stone towers on Route 1A (Ocean Road), Narragansett. **Season:** Year-round. **Admission:** Free. **Telephone:** (401) 783-7121.

SCARBOROUGH STATE BEACH. Directions: Located on Route 1A in Narragansett. **Season:** Formal season from end of June through Labor Day. **Admission:** Charged. **Telephone:** (401) 277-2632.

SOUTH COUNTY MUSEUM. Directions: Located on Canonchet Farm, off Route 1A, just north of The Towers. Enter through the parking lot opposite the large beach pavilion. Explain that you are going to the museum and you won't have to pay the beach parking fee. **Season:** April through October (weekends only in April and May, September and October). **Admission:** Charged; group discounts. **Telephone:** (401) 783-5400.

M/V *SOUTHLAND*. Directions: Departures from State Pier in Galilee. **Season:** Memorial Day through Labor Day. **Admission:** Charged. **Telephone:** (401) 783-2954.

EAST MATUNUCK STATE BEACH. Directions: Located in South Kingston. Take Route 1A south from Narragansett and follow signs to beach. **Season:** Formal season from end of June through Labor Day. **Admission:** Parking fee. **Telephone:** (401) 277-2632.

JIM'S DOCKSIDE. Directions: Take Route 1A south from Narragansett, turning off at sign for Jerusalem. Follow Succotash Road right into town. Bear right at center of town (where you have to make a choice). Follow road for 2 miles. Jim's is on the right. **Season:** May through October. **Admission:** Free. **Telephone:** (401) 783-2050.

For further information or restaurant and lodging suggestions, write to the Narragansett Chamber of Commerce, The Towers, Ocean Road/Route 1A, Narragansett, RI 02882.

MASSACHUSETTS

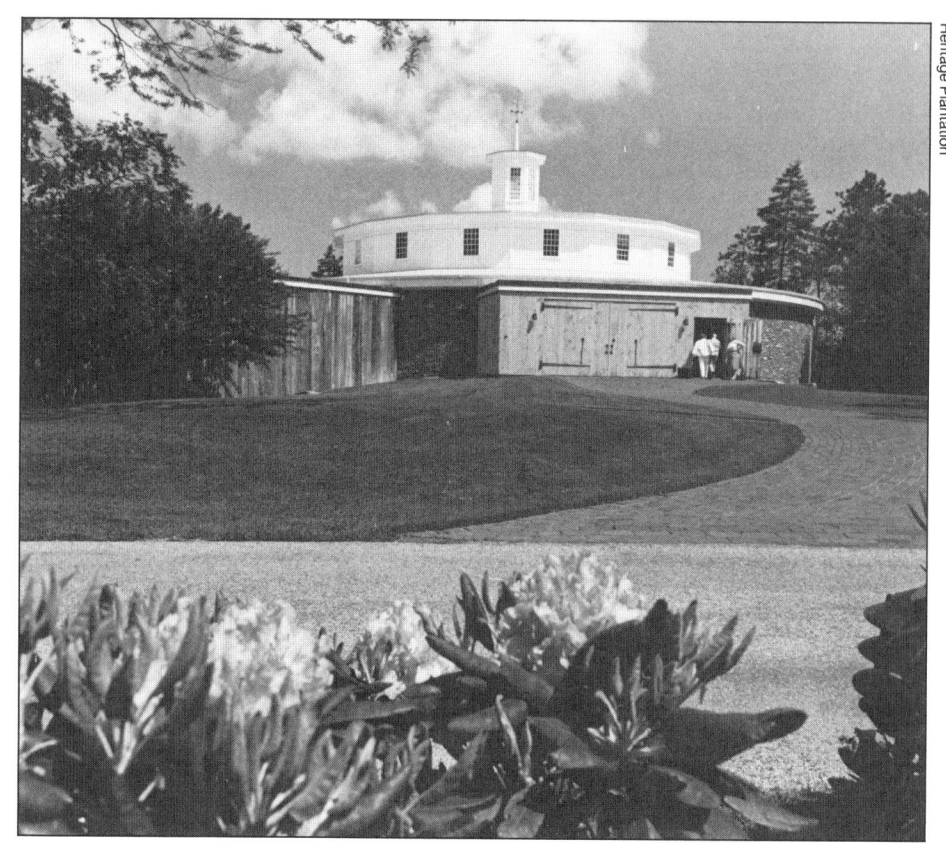

The old Shaker round barn, a prominent feature of the 76-acre Heritage Plantation of Sandwich, houses a handsome collection of antique cars, including a 1915 Stutz Bearcat and a 1931 Duesenberg.

Sandwich

Sandwich, Cape Cod's oldest town, got its start in 1637 when Plymouth Colony granted to "Ten Men from Saugus" the right to settle enough land for "three score families." Today Sandwich is best known for its most famous native son, children's author Thornton W. Burgess, and its most famous industry, glassmaking. If you read the Mother West Wind stories to your children (or if your own parents read them to you), you'll probably feel a wave of nostalgia as you visit places associated with Burgess and the characters he created.

Thornton Burgess (1874–1965) spent most of his life in Sandwich. A naturalist and conservationist, he immortalized the lovely stream- and pond-studded woodlands where he grew up and played as a child in the pages of the more than 170 books and 15,000 stories he produced during a career that spanned five decades. As a boy, Burgess worked as a messenger for a mail-order pond lily business and spent much of his time roaming the woods in East Sandwich. Later drawing upon his memories, he brought to print and radio stories about Mother West Wind, Peter Rabbit, and their many friends.

Burgess's work and memory are perpetuated by the Thornton W. Burgess Society, which operates the **Green Briar Nature Center and Jam Kitchen** in East Sandwich and the **Thornton W. Burgess Museum** in Sandwich Center. Founded to "inspire reverence for wildlife and concern for the natural environment," the society sponsors a rich assortment of programs, including a series of guided Saturday morning nature walks and midweek evening slide lectures. Also offered is a wide selection of single-session adult natural history classes, field trips, and craft programs, covering subjects from bird watching and basket making to jam cookery and canoeing. For a schedule of events, write to Green Briar Nature Center, East Sandwich, MA 02537.

Whether or not you enroll in a walk or a workshop, you'll want to visit the center, where you can admire a wildflower garden containing more than a hundred varieties. No matter what the season, you can enjoy a half-hour hike through the Briar Patch, taking care not to trip on the roots that crisscross the narrow, hilly, but well-maintained trail.

Inside the nature center you can tour the Jam Kitchen, where jams, jellies, and preserves are made the old-fashioned way — without preservatives and additives — just as they have been for more than eighty years. Twenty gas burners run down the center of the spacious blue-and-white kitchen, where ladles, sieves, and measuring cups hang from wall hooks. You're likely to come upon volunteers busily labeling jars and peeling peaches over large enamel basins. Other workers check the jams "cooking" in the solar cookers. If you participate in a jam-making workshop, you'll have a sample to take home. If you don't, you can buy some tasty remembrances in the gift shop. Choose from classics such as beach plum jelly and raspberry jam, or opt for something more exotic like lemon-lime marmalade.

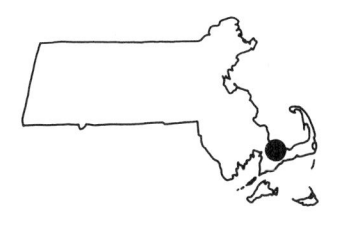

If you have a grandchild along, try to schedule your visit for a summer afternoon. Story hour is at 1:30 P.M.

Perched on the edge of Shawme Lake, the **Thornton W. Burgess Museum** contains the largest known collection of Burgess's writings and a wealth of original drawings by Harrison Cady, who illustrated Burgess's stories for fifty years. Cady's work is characterized by whimsically dressed animals whose faces reflect human emotions. There are also several natural history exhibits relating to the author's life and work. If you have a grandchild along, try to schedule your visit for a summer afternoon. Story hour is at 1:30 P.M., Tuesday through Saturday, in July and August, complete with a live animal visitor. In addition, geese, ducks, and swans often pay impromptu visits to the museum lawn, looking for a handout.

At the **Sandwich Glass Museum** the focus is on the superb collection of locally manufactured nineteenth-century glass, displayed together with associated historical materials. In the "factory room" you'll see original equipment used by the Boston & Sandwich Company, one of the earliest of several glass factories to set up business in Sandwich, incorporating in 1826. (The factory continued to make blown and pressed glass, plain and decorated, for sixty-three years.) Old photographs, glassmaking tools and materials, and a diorama depicting the manufacturing process are among the displays.

With plenty of light and generous arrangements of fresh flowers, the museum offers an ideal setting for displays that vary from a collection of children's toys from the 1830s (miniature glass decanters, goblets, and pitchers) to a window filled with shelves of mid-nineteenth-century dolphin candlesticks (rated as among the most characteristic pieces of Sandwich glass). One entire wall is filled with pressed glass compotes, lamps, vases, bar bottles, and salts in a rainbow of colors. You'll also see scent bottles, canes, letter seals, paperweights, and novelties such as a bear-shaped pomade jar, all made from glass. Another museum room houses artifacts belonging to early Sandwich residents, and paintings, furniture, maps, and photographs associated with the town's history are displayed throughout the museum's eleven galleries.

Several other places to visit are within walking distance of the museum. If you're a doll fancier, get ready for another wave of nostalgia as you enter the **Yesteryears Doll Museum,** located in the former First Parish Meetinghouse. Most of the treasures are exhibited in glass cases suspended across old pews.

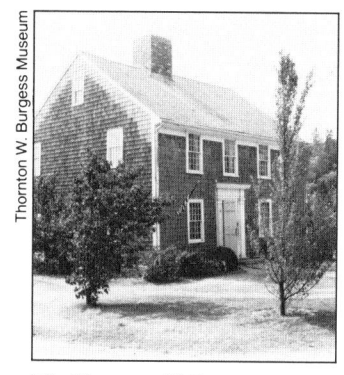

The Thornton W. Burgess Museum contains many original drawings by Harrison Cady, who illustrated Burgess's children's stories for fifty years.

There are famous dolls such as Mme. Alexander's Dionne Quintuplets and Ideal's Shirley Temple, not to mention dolls you may have given to your own children, such as Hasbro's early G.I. Joe or Mattel's Barbie. Make certain to seek out Bye-Lo Baby, the first doll modeled after a real baby. The woman who donated her to the museum spent a full year (1923) peddling Barnett's vanilla extract to earn money to purchase this precious possession.

Period dollhouse rooms reflecting changing tastes in interior design are also displayed. One late nineteenth-century scene is chock-full of the heavy oak pieces so popular during the late Victorian period. Another represents a milliner's shop, complete with dozens of tiny bonnets for fashion-conscious dolls to choose from. You'll also see dolls from every corner of the world — including milk carriers from Spain, Yugoslavia, China, and Switzerland — as well as paper dolls, early toys, and doll beds.

The museum shop sells antique dolls along with reproductions of old toys; patterns; doll wigs, shoes, and stockings; and dollhouse furnishings. If your childhood doll is in need of a face-lift or other restoration, bring her along for a doll doctor's estimate.

For quite another taste of history, take a ten-minute tour of **Hoxie House,** a fully restored and furnished late seventeenth-century saltbox, once home to a minister, his wife, and their thirteen children. Your guide will point out architectural features such as the windows made of hand-blown glass framed in lead and original furnishings such as the hired hand's bed that opens flat, forerunner of today's convertible sofa. Up on the second floor, which you're free to explore independently, watch for the unusual wooden bonnet box.

Still within easy walking distance of the Glass Museum is **Thomas Dexter's Grist Mill,** where waterfowl glide across the surface of the millpond. Seventy percent of the original structure, built from 1640 to 1646, is still intact, and water from the pond continues to drive the large wooden water wheel just as it did three centuries ago. Corn is ground between the two huge millstones, each weighing over a thousand pounds. The mill produces more than sixteen thousand two-pound bags of cornmeal each summer, and you can purchase some to take home to transform into Indian pudding, spoon bread, corn bread, or pancakes.

Thornton Burgess has left his mark here, too. One of his verses hangs on the mill wall:

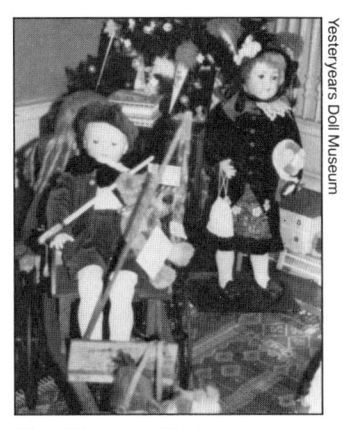

This Victorian Christmas scene is but a small sampling of the treasures waiting to be discovered at the Yesteryears Doll Museum.

MASSACHUSETTS / 43

God bless the miller and his wheel!
God bless the merry till!
As long ago in Unison,
I hear them singing still.
And he who thinks that melody
May think or do no ill.

While you are in the center of town, duck into the **First Church of Christ,** built in 1847 in the architectural tradition of Christopher Wren, complete with soaring spire. Be sure to take a look at the Captain Adolph Bell; cast in 1675, it is reputed to be the oldest church bell in America. Also on display is a 1715 pulpit Bible and the antique pipe organ built the same year as the church.

Just a short drive from the center of town, you'll come to **Heritage Plantation of Sandwich**. You can easily spend half a day here, traveling the well-tended paths that meander past gardens, through woodlands, and along the banks of Upper Shawme Lake. These areas provide a home for more than a thousand varieties of trees, shrubs, and flowers. There's a holly dell, a day lily display garden (in bloom mid-July through the first week of August), and a huge rhododendron display (mid-May through mid-June). The seventy-six-acre plantation is also a museum housing a diverse collection of Americana. Exhibit buildings are spread far apart, but an open-air shuttle bus makes frequent trips around the grounds, offering free, convenient transportation.

Begin your visit with a stop at the reproduction Shaker round barn to ogle the handsomely preserved vintage and antique cars. Don't miss the shiny yellow Stutz Bearcat (1915) with its padded black leather bucket seats, just as much a symbol of the Jazz Age as hip flasks and raccoon coats. As a placard explains, "The Bearcat was not only romantic, it was tough." The canary yellow and pistachio Duesenberg (1931) with dark green upholstery isn't hard to take either. For even more nostalgia, movies featuring early film stars and their exotic cars are screened daily in the adjoining theater.

At the military museum building you'll see two thousand hand-painted military miniatures, along with a collection of antique firearms. The museum also houses a small but noteworthy collection of Native American art and artifacts, including an intricate mid-nineteenth-century headdress made of eagle feathers, horsehair, porcupine quills, and ribbon, and suspended in a glass case, looking for all the world like an enormous, delicate insect.

Be sure to take a look at the Captain Adolph Bell; cast in 1675, it is reputed to be the oldest church bell in America.

Two thousand hand-painted miniatures and numerous antique firearms enrich the collection in Heritage Plantation's military building.

The art museum features displays of scrimshaw, weather vanes, cigar store figures, bird carvings, landscape and genre paintings, and Western art. The lower level contains an outstanding collection of Currier and Ives prints. Between 1834 and 1907, the New York firm of Nathaniel Currier and James Merritt Ives produced approximately ten million prints, which sold for twenty cents to three dollars apiece. The subjects of these examples include familiar themes: a winter sleigh ride, cows returning from pasture, a baseball game, trolling for bluefish. When you finish admiring the artwork, your ears will draw you upstairs to the glassed-in rotunda, where a restored 1912 carousel, complete with bejeweled wooden animals, circles to period music. You're welcome to climb aboard!

Heritage Plantation has a gift shop, but it does not offer food service. Pets and picnics are not permitted on the grounds, but there is a pleasant picnic area just outside the main gate.

If you want to assemble a last-minute picnic, head for **Sandwich's Sandwiches,** an informal lunch shop tucked into a petite storefront. The service is strictly do-it-yourself, but you can pull up a stool at one of the four barrel-shaped tables if you want to eat on the premises. The staff will be happy to put up a box lunch if you want to eat elsewhere.

The theme here is "create your own sandwich," and there are plenty of ingredients from which to choose. Start with one of the basics, such as baked ham or seafood salad. Then select from eight types of bread before turning your attention to the ten toppings (sprouts to cucumbers, mushrooms to pickles), seven cheeses, and nine spreads (Pommery mustard to hot pepper, herb mayonnaise to chutney). Or choose one of the daily specials listed on the old-fashioned wall slate, a crisp salad or some home-

Your ears will draw you upstairs, where a restored 1912 carousel circles to period music. You're welcome to climb aboard!

made soup. For dessert choose from homemade cookies, carrot cake, brownies, and, sometimes, raspberry-almond bars.

If you have an insatiable sweet tooth, you'll want to drop in next door at **Carousel Candies,** where the proprietor often stations herself near the window, dipping chocolates between customers. Another window showcases the shop's namesake, a miniature wooden carousel complete with horse, goose, rooster, and pig. The baby blue and coral pink decor creates a fanciful ambiance, where it's lots of fun to choose from dozens of varieties of chocolates and fudges, creams and caramels, macadamia nut "caterpillars" and splendid almond butter crunch.

The shop also stocks novelty items such as chocolate computers; brown-and-white chocolate pandas; tiny seashell-shaped candies in delicate shades of pink, orange, blue, and green; and a wonderful chocolate box filled with chocolate-dipped fruits. There is a good selection of diabetic chocolates, including almond bark, peanut butter truffles, and pecan-raisin clusters. What more pleasant way to end a busy day than to nibble on fresh candy as you make your way home.

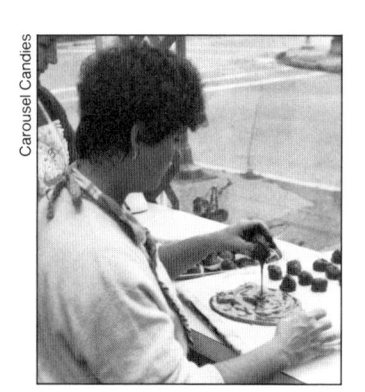

Hand-dipped chocolates are a house specialty at Carousel Candies.

ACCESS

SANDWICH. Follow Route 3 south, crossing the Cape Cod Canal over the Sagamore Bridge. From the bridge, follow Route 6 (Mid-Cape Highway) east. Take exit 2, following Route 130 north into Sandwich.

GREEN BRIAR NATURE CENTER AND JAM KITCHEN. Directions: From the center of Sandwich, follow Route 6A east about 2 miles, in the direction of East Sandwich. Turn right on Discovery Hill Road, following signs to center. **Season:** Year-round; jam making from June through December. **Admission:** Free. **Telephone:** (617) 888-6870.

THORNTON W. BURGESS MUSEUM. Directions: Located on Water Street in the center of Sandwich. **Season:** Year-round. **Admission:** Donation requested. **Telephone:** (617) 888-6870.

SANDWICH GLASS MUSEUM. Directions: Located across from the town hall in the center of town. **Season:** April through October. November, December, February, and March, Wednesday through Sunday only. **Admission:** Charged. **Telephone:** (617) 888-0251. **Note:** Handicapped accessible.

YESTERYEARS DOLL MUSEUM. Directions: Located at the corner of Main and River streets in the center of town. **Season:** Mid-May through October. **Admission:**

Charged; senior discount. Group rates available (call ahead). **Telephone:** (617) 888-1711. **Note:** Exhibits are located up one flight of stairs.

HOXIE HOUSE. Directions: Located on Water Street in the center of town. **Season:** Mid-June through mid-October. **Admission:** Charged. **Telephone:** (617) 888-1173.

THOMAS DEXTER'S GRIST MILL. Directions: Located on Water Street in the center of town, adjacent to the Thornton W. Burgess Museum. **Season:** Mid-June through mid-October. **Admission:** Charged. **Telephone:** (617) 888-1173.

FIRST CHURCH OF CHRIST. Directions: Located on Main Street in the center of town. **Season:** Year-round. **Admission:** Free. **Telephone:** (617) 888-0434.

HERITAGE PLANTATION OF SANDWICH. Directions: Follow Route 6A to Route 130 south, veering right at fork in road, then follow signs to Heritage Plantation, located at the intersection of Grove and Pine streets. **Season:** Mid-May through late October. **Admission:** Charged. **Telephone:** (617) 888-3300. **Note:** Many exhibits are located on ground level, with entry ramps located next to stairs into buildings. Handicapped-accessible rest rooms.

SANDWICH'S SANDWICHES. Directions: Located on Jarves Street at Russell's Corner (junction of Jarves Street and Route 6A). **Season:** Year-round. **Admission:** Free. **Telephone:** (617) 888-1221.

CAROUSEL CANDIES. Directions: Located at 132 Route 6A, next to Sandwich's Sandwiches. **Season:** Year-round. **Admission:** Free. **Telephone:** (617) 888-7000.

For further information or restaurant and lodging suggestions, contact the Cape Cod Chamber of Commerce, U.S. Route 6 and Massachusetts Route 132, Hyannis, MA 02601. Telephone: (617) 362-3225.

Boston

When restlessness sets in, no matter what the season, think Boston. When you start to feel bored, isolated, and in need of some excitement, remember Boston. When you're hungry for a slice of history, music, or theater; classy shops and restaurants; or a good competitive sporting event, fill up on Boston. And do it your way. If you worry about getting lost in a strange city, take a bus tour. Like to tour at your own pace but without the hassle of driving? Buy an all-day trolley ticket. A guided walking trip or a narrated harbor cruise offer two other options for discovering the city some call the "Hub of the Universe."

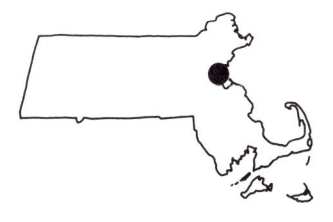

Feast on the wealth of cultural and recreational opportunities that flow from the city like fruit from a horn of plenty.

Few cities rival Boston as a place of American historical significance.

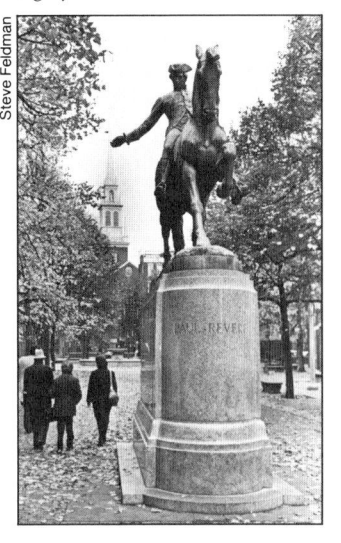

It would be easy to write a whole book describing this vibrant city's historic attractions, museums, performing arts institutions, educational facilities, and eclectic neighborhoods. Since it is impossible to be comprehensive here, our tack is to suggest a "Beginner's Boston." Interpret "beginner" to mean novice sightseer. It doesn't mean that you've never been to Boston before. You may even travel to the city frequently on business or to shop, but not to sightsee. Just as many people never visit the important sites in their own hometown until they entertain a visitor from far away, many of us have never taken the time to check out our own urban backyard the way out-of-towners do. When it comes to touring Boston, that situation is a pleasure to remedy.

If you are not familiar with the "Hub" — a genuine "beginner" — these suggestions will help you become comfortable exploring the city. Just remember, the advice here is only a start. We want to give you a sense of Boston's history and of her geographic layout. Once that has been accomplished, we hope you will feast on the wealth of cultural and recreational opportunities that flow from the city like fruit from a horn of plenty.

An excellent way to key in to "what's happening" is to stop by the **Greater Boston Convention and Visitors Bureau** in the Prudential Center. This is the place to pick up brochures, maps, and schedules. You'll get the lowdown on both permanent and visiting attractions, along with personal advice on how to use your time in the city to best advantage, taking into account your tastes and interests. Come loaded with questions; you'll be rewarded with insightful, informative answers.

A great way to get an overview of the city is to hike **The Freedom Trail,** a walking tour that ties together many of the places, personalities, and events that played a part in the colonial era and the American Revolution. The trail winds through the city from Boston Common to the Charlestown Navy Yard, and it is marked by a broad red line painted on the sidewalk. A leisurely walk covering all sixteen sites along the trail will take about three hours.

Boston Common, where you can pick up a trail guide at the Boston Common Visitor Information Center, is the oldest public park in the country. From the Common travel to the "new" State House, designed by eighteenth-century architect Charles Bulfinch (free tours available) and then to the Park Street Church, where William Lloyd Garrison gave his first antislavery address in 1829. Next to the

The USS Constitution Museum features this exact scale model of "Old Ironsides," the world's oldest warship still afloat.

church is the Granary Burying Ground, final resting place of illustrious Americans John Hancock, Samuel Adams, and Paul Revere. Continue on to King's Chapel, the site of the first public school in the country; the Old Corner Bookstore (where literary greats including Longfellow and Hawthorne once gathered); the Old South Meeting House; the Old State House; the Boston Massacre site; Faneuil Hall; the Paul Revere House; the Old North Church; Copp's Hill Burying Ground; the USS *Constitution*; and Bunker Hill Monument. Many of the sites are open to the public (see ACCESS section). Allow extra time for those you wish to visit.

If you take your time to enjoy every aspect of the trail, from the shopping and lively street entertainment at Quincy Market (adjacent to Faneuil Hall) to the exhibits at the Paul Revere House and from the USS *Constitution* Museum to the multimedia presentations at the Old South Meeting House and the Bunker Hill Pavilion (near the USS *Constitution*), you'll need at least two full days.

There are several ways to undertake the Freedom Trail. If you want to conserve your energy, if you are not particularly comfortable in large cities, or if you worry about getting lost, try a guided bus trip. **Brush Hill Tours** conducts a three-and-a-quarter-hour tour that takes you past Beacon Hill, Government Center, Faneuil Hall, the waterfront, and Fenway Park. You'll travel to the Charlestown Navy Yard, home of the USS *Constitution*, the oldest commissioned naval warship in the country, and you'll get a glimpse of the swan boats gliding smoothly over the duck pond in the Public Garden. The tour

Boston Common is the oldest public park in the country.

also passes fancy Copley Place, an upscale shopper's mecca, and Copley Square, where venerable Trinity Church casts its reflection in the glass walls of the soaring John Hancock Tower. You then cross the Charles River to Cambridge and pass by academic legends Harvard and MIT. Your guide will provide a running commentary throughout the tour, describing the historical events and contemporary activities that make Boston a special city.

While the major part of the trip is spent on the bus, two stops allow you to get out and visit the site (at your own expense), take a walk and pick up a snack, or just stay comfortably seated on the bus. The first is at **The Boston Tea Party Ship and Museum,** where you can relive the evening of December 16, 1773, when the colonists protested British taxation without representation by hurling nine thousand pounds of tea overboard. The small museum explores the causes and effects of this rowdy rebellion and uses films, historical documents, and artifacts such as an original tea chest to capture the mood of pre-Revolutionary Boston.

Be sure to take a few minutes to figure out where your politics would have placed you back then. To determine whether you fall in the patriot or loyalist camp, just fill out the brief quiz indicating your degree of agreement or disagreement with statements such as "Government is more often the enemy than the friend."

Continue on to board the *Brig Beaver II,* a full-size working replica of one of the original Tea Party ships. Feeling cantankerous? Work off some of your energy by tossing a bale of tea overboard into the harbor below. (It's attached to the boat by a rope so you can haul it up afterward, but heaving it into the drink still provides a very satisfying feeling.) Do be aware that there are steps involved in visiting the museum and the brig, particularly if you want to go below decks.

If you would rather remain on dry land, you can head over to nearby **Museum Wharf,** home of the Children's Museum and the Computer Museum, which you may want to return to later when you have more time. Just aim for the giant milk bottle. In warm weather the milk bottle is a food stand, selling ice cream, salads, yogurt, and other snacks. The wharf has lots of benches where you can eat or just observe the activity on the water.

The second stop is at the Charlestown Navy Yard. The line to the **USS *Constitution*** is often tedious in the summer and fall, involving an hour or

Feeling cantankerous? Work off some of your energy by tossing a bale of tea overboard into the harbor below.

more wait before you can climb the steep gangplank to the upper deck. The bus company does not guarantee enough time to visit the ship if the line is long. If you do board, be aware that you'll need to navigate ladders if you want to go below. There's also a lot of stooping and bending involved in getting through the narrow passageways. You'll pass cannon with names like Sweet Sue and Raging Eagle, and you'll peer into the purser's quarters (so cramped that he'd just toss a mattress across his desk when it was time to go to sleep), the surgeon's room, and lots of other nooks and crannies.

At this second stop you might choose instead to view "The Whites of Their Eyes" at the **Bunker Hill Pavilion,** located two hundred yards from "Old Ironsides" but not formally part of the Freedom Trail. A multimedia presentation is shown in a comfortable theater with screens all around. Slides, music, and special effects re-create the drama of the first major battle of the Revolution. Or you can visit the **USS *Constitution* Museum,** where you'll see historic maritime paintings and artifacts along with exhibits designed to give a sense of what life was like for an eighteenth-century seaman.

If you prefer to travel alone instead of as part of a group, you can combine the best of both worlds by buying a ticket good for a full day of travel aboard **Beantown Trolleys**. These reproduction Victorian era trolleys, with their wood-and-brass decor, are fun to ride and can save you a lot of walking. The driver provides narration, too, so you'll get the information you need to enjoy the sites. The trolley makes six stops — at Boston Common, Copley Square, the USS *Constitution* and museum, Quincy Market, and a couple of hotels — and you can get on and off as often as you please during the course of the day. The stops put most of Boston's major attractions within easy walking distance.

When you buy your ticket, you'll be given a map. You might consider getting an early start, riding the trolley the entire route (one-and-a-half-hour tour), and marking on your map the places you would like to return to via trolley later in the day. This arrangement provides both an orientation to the city and the opportunity to pursue your own interests independently and at your own pace.

Another way to get oriented is to view the city from 740 feet off the ground. Take the express elevator to the sixtieth floor of New England's tallest building and you'll find yourself in the **John Hancock Observatory**. The panorama of the city,

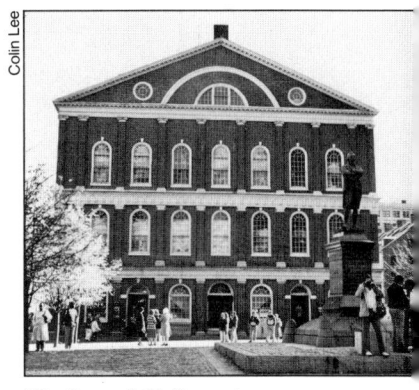

The Faneuil Hall stop is a highlight on Boston's popular Freedom Trail walking tour.

MASSACHUSETTS / 51

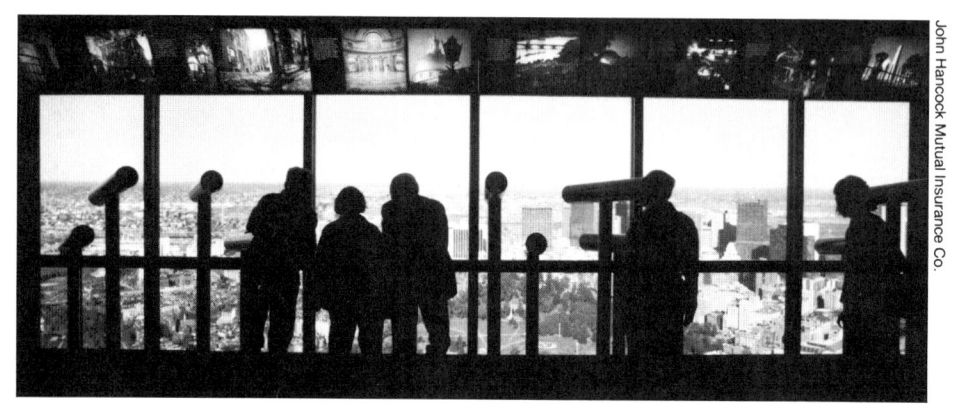

From the John Hancock Observatory, 740 feet up in New England's tallest building, the view of Boston and surroundings is spectacular.

stretching out on all sides of the glassed-in area, is the big draw. You'll spot the gold-domed State House on Beacon Hill and the sailboats on the Charles. Far in the distance, on a clear day, you can see the White Mountains of New Hampshire.

The observatory houses some intriguing exhibits, too, including "Boston 1775," a sound and light show played out on a giant relief map. There's also a quick-moving film that hones in on the people, places, and traditions that make Boston the city it is today. And there are carpeted tiers where you can sit and admire the cityscape below while listening to a tape in which the late architectural historian Walter Muir Whitehill describes the changes that have occurred in the city's skyline since its early days.

Should you be a devoted walker with a keen interest in architecture, you might want to take a guided city walk sponsored by **Boston By Foot**. These trips run whether two (you and the guide) or twenty show up. The guides are trained volunteers with a contagious enthusiasm for their city, and you may well feel more like a friend than a paying customer. Boston By Foot offers four different regularly scheduled walks, each lasting an hour and a half.

The "Heart of the Freedom Trail" tour covers nine designated Freedom Trail sites, including the Old State House, where the Declaration of Independence was first read in Boston, Faneuil Hall, and Quincy Market. The "Beacon Hill" tour focuses on the architecture of Charles Bulfinch and his followers, as evidenced in the elegant townhouses of Louisburg Square. The "Copley Square in Back Bay" tour emphasizes Trinity Church, Old South Church, the Boston Public Library, and some of the nearby mansions that are also part of this nineteenth-century neighborhood. Boston has a long and colorful ethnic history, and the "North End" tour is a good introduction to the city's oldest neighborhood, now an Italian enclave, where you'll be tempted by festive bakeries and markets as you weave your way through the narrow streets en route to landmarks such as the Old North Church, the Paul Revere House, and Copp's Hill Burying Ground.

Still another way to get a feel for the city is to cruise her waters, surely a fitting way to get acquainted with a historic seaport. **Boston Harbor Cruises** offers a ninety-minute narrated harbor cruise. You'll learn about local history and legend as your captain points out the site of the Boston Tea Party, the spire of the Old North Church, and other landmarks. You'll also find out about the evolution of the waterfront itself, from colonial to contemporary times, and you'll get a look at the Boston Harbor Islands as you move into the outer harbor. (For complete details on visiting the islands, see *Island Hopping in New England*, published by Yankee Books.)

If you prefer to combine your nautical adventure with some land-bound sightseeing, take the "Constitution Shuttle," a shorter version of the cruise described above, with the added option that you can disembark at the Charlestown Navy Yard for a visit to "Old Ironsides" and the USS *Constitution* Museum before reboarding for the return trip to Long Wharf at Boston Harbor. The trip takes about fifteen minutes in each direction. Allow forty-five minutes for the complete circuit if you choose to stay aboard straight through. Forty-minute lunchtime cruises (bring your own brown bag) and ninety-minute sunset cruises are also offered.

You'll be tempted by festive bakeries and markets as you weave your way through the narrow streets en route to landmarks.

ACCESS

GREATER BOSTON CONVENTION AND VISITORS BUREAU. Directions: Located in the Prudential Center. **Season:** Year-round. **Admission:** Free. **Telephone:** (617) 536-4100.

THE FREEDOM TRAIL. Directions: Pick up trail map and guide at the Boston Common Visitor Information Center near the Park Street subway station at Boston Common. **Season:** Year-round. **Admission:** The following sites charge entrance fees; those followed by "$" offer senior discounts (and are free to those holding a Golden Age Passport): Old South Meeting House ($), Old State House ($), Paul Revere House ($), USS *Constitution* Museum ($), Bunker Hill Monument. **Telephone:** (800) 858-0200.

BRUSH HILL TOURS. Directions: Ticket office located at the Sheraton Boston Hotel, 39 Dalton Street, adjacent to

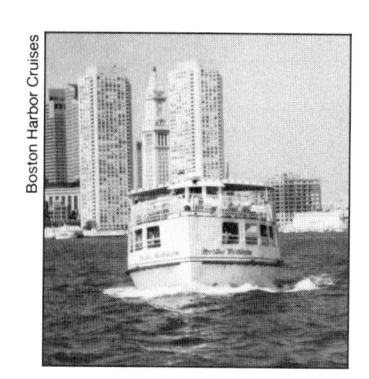

Boston Harbor Cruises features ninety-minute seagoing tours of historic Boston Harbor and the outlying islands.

the Prudential Center. **Season:** Year-round. **Admission:** Charged. **Telephone:** (617) 287-1900.

THE BOSTON TEA PARTY SHIP AND MUSEUM. Directions: Located at the Congress Street Bridge. **Season:** Year-round. **Admission:** Charged; senior discount. **Telephone:** (617) 338-1773.

USS *CONSTITUTION*. Directions: Ship is docked at the Charlestown Navy Yard. **Season:** Year-round. **Admission:** Free. **Telephone:** (617) 426-1812.

BUNKER HILL PAVILION. Directions: Located about 200 yards from the USS *Constitution*. **Season:** Year-round. **Admission:** Charged; senior discount. **Telephone:** (617) 241-7575.

USS *CONSTITUTION* MUSEUM. Directions: Located in the Charlestown Navy Yard. **Season:** Year-round. **Admission:** Charged; senior discount. **Telephone:** (617) 426-1812.

BEANTOWN TROLLEYS. Directions: Purchase tickets and board trolley at the Boston Common Visitor Information Center or any of the other stops. **Season:** Year-round. **Admission:** Charged. **Telephone:** (617) 287-1900.

JOHN HANCOCK OBSERVATORY. Directions: John Hancock Tower is located at Copley Square. Observatory ticket office is at the corner of the building at Trinity Place and St. James Avenue. **Season:** Year-round. **Admission:** Charged; senior discount. **Telephone:** (617) 247-1977.

BOSTON BY FOOT. Directions: Each tour begins at a different location. Tickets can be purchased at BOSTIX at Faneuil Hall Marketplace or directly from the guide at the meeting place. Telephone for a leaflet detailing times and places. **Season:** May through October. **Admission:** Charged. **Telephone:** (617) 367-2345.

BOSTON HARBOR CRUISES. Directions: Ticket center is located at 1 Long Wharf, near Atlantic Avenue at the base of State Street, one block from Quincy Market. **Season:** Peak season is June 15 through Labor Day. Reduced schedule in spring and fall. **Admission:** Charged; senior discount. **Telephone:** (617) 227-4321.

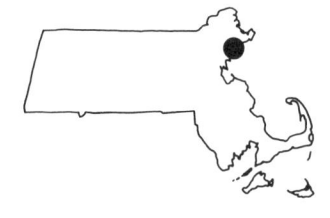

Salem

A robust seaport during the height of the clipper ship days, scene of the infamous seventeenth-century witch trials, and home of author Nathaniel Hawthorne, Salem is filled with stories that illuminate early American maritime, literary, social, and domestic history. With fine museums, a lively harbor, and attractive places to eat and shop, Salem is a pleasure to explore. Plan to stay a night or two or, if you have only a day, tell yourself that you'll be back soon.

Because there is so much to see in Salem and because some of the attractions are a fair distance from one another, you might want to avoid the inconvenience of moving your car from one spot to another by leaving it in the outdoor pay parking lot behind the Witch Museum or the indoor pay lot across from East India Square and the Peabody Museum. Then buy a ticket entitling you to all-day shuttle service aboard the **Salem Trolley**. Named "The Hawthorne," this trackless, motorized, thirty-four-passenger vehicle is built to resemble a turn-of-the-century trolley. Painted red, it has etched-glass windows, hardwood interior trim, and a real San Francisco cable car gong. The trolley runs in a loop pattern all day long. You might want to stay on for one complete loop, which will provide you with a narrated tour of forty points of interest. Or you can take your tour in bits and pieces, getting on and off at the twelve stops, located near major points of interest throughout the city.

The **Peabody Museum of Salem,** the oldest continually operating museum in the country, originated in 1799 with the formation of the East India Marine Society. Such organizations, formed to assist the widows and children of deceased members

Plan to stay a night or two or, if you have only a day, tell yourself that you'll be back soon.

Many exquisite maritime items, such as this sextant, grace the collection of Salem's Peabody Museum.

MASSACHUSETTS / 55

(many of them lost at sea) and to collect information that would make navigation safer, were not uncommon in the eighteenth and nineteenth centuries. What was unique about the East India Marine Society was the expression in its charter of the desire "to form a Museum of natural and artificial curiosities." Membership in this particular society was limited to Salem sea captains who had sailed in the area of the Cape of Good Hope or Cape Horn. It was these captains who brought back to Salem the artifacts that form the nucleus of the museum's collections covering maritime history, natural history, ethnology, archaeology, and Asian export art.

Here you will see exhibits that vary from detailed dioramas illustrating the early days on the Salem waterfront (complete with miniature kegs of rum and a tiny wharf rat) to a statue of the Hawaiian war god Kukailimoku, one of only three such statues in the world. Exhibits include many fine examples of Chinese export porcelain and other decorative wares brought back from the Orient, along with clothing, weapons, tools, and utensils from the South Pacific islands. The maritime collection includes figureheads, scrimshaw, sailors' artifacts, paintings, portraits, navigational and fishing gear, and ship models. There's even a full-size reconstruction of the Master's Saloon of *Cleopatra's Barge*, America's first ocean-going yacht, built in 1816.

In addition to permanent and visiting exhibits, the museum sponsors an extensive schedule of special activities. (Call or write ahead for a calendar of events.) A gallery talk on ship models includes a tour of models in the museum, with an explanation of the varying roles they have played in different societies. You learn that this is the oldest form of marine art and that while the models' function is now primarily decorative, they used to be used as burial offerings and given as gifts to the gods.

The museum faces the Essex Street Mall, a pleasant pedestrian walkway paved in brick and cobblestones. It is lined with attractive stores that you may wish to explore, but even if you don't feel like shopping, do take a few minutes to admire the East India Square Fountain. Designed to symbolize Salem's historic relationship with the Orient, the fountain features a towering Japanese gate from which water pours into a pool that represents Salem harbor. There are two levels of stone in the pool, one that delineates Salem's shoreline in the 1700s and another that shows its contours today, with large portions of the harbor filled in.

The Peabody Museum of Salem, the oldest continually operating museum in the country, originated in 1799.

Just a block away, at the **Essex Institute,** you can learn more about the evolution of Salem's history by visiting a trio of historic homes, chronicling changes in domestic life through three centuries. The institute also has its own museum, well worth a visit if you do not have the time or energy for the hour-and-a-quarter tour through the three houses. Here you'll find exhibits of furnished rooms, including an early New England kitchen (c. 1750), an 1815 vintage bedroom, and a parlor dating to about 1825. There is also an exhibit focusing on the industrial history of Essex County (where Salem is located). Another display, a history of cutlery, explains that the spoon was the only tool used for eating in the seventeenth-century Essex County home, if any utensil was used at all. This was supplemented in the eighteenth century by the wide-blade knife, which, along with the two- or three-tine fork, was used for cutting meat but not for eating.

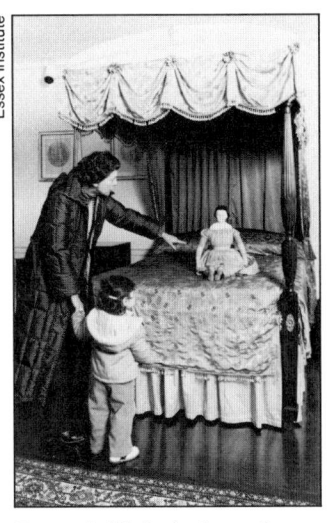

Domestic life is the focus of exhibits at the Essex Institute's three historic houses.

The house tour begins in the **John Ward House** (c. 1684), which predates the famous witchcraft trials. A simple dwelling, the house was moved to this site in 1910 from Prison Lane, two blocks away. In its original location, opposite the jail, it was used to house accused witches while they awaited trial. The ceilings are low, the beams heavy, the walls covered with whitewash, and the windows done in leaded diamond-shaped panes. Furnishings are sparse and simple, but they do include an early bed with a wooden key for tightening the rope springs, a practice that gives us the expression "sleep tight."

One room of the house has been set up to represent a nineteenth-century apothecary shop, complete with bloodletting devices, tall glass jars of medicines, and a ship's wooden medical chest with drawers labeled "serpentaria," "spongia," and other ominous-sounding names. Pass through the weaving room, with its flax and cotton spinning wheels and huge wooden floor loom, and into the "cent" shop, a predecessor of the nearly defunct twentieth-century dime store. Wives of men at sea often ran such shops to supplement their income, selling everything from their own handwork to playing cards painted by their children. This one is even set up to serve as a post office, but your guide will explain that in those days the person who *received* the letter paid the postage. If you didn't pick up your mail within a given time, the postmaster would publicly post it for all to read.

Next on the tour is the Georgian style **Crowninshield–Bentley House** (c. 1727), which belonged to a series of men who sailed ships out of Salem. Two parlors illustrate the evolution of home furnishing and decoration. One is very simple, furnished 1727 style, while the other is quite elegant, remodeled in 1794. The kitchen contains lots of interesting equipment, such as an iron used for putting a ruffle or flounce into a dress while it was being worn. Upstairs the bedrooms are furnished with canopy beds, early washstands and commodes, a fine chest on chest, and many other period pieces.

The final stop is the brick, neoclassical style **Gardner-Pingree House,** which reflects the increasing affluence of a successful importer who made his fortune trading in the Orient. The house has exceptional woodcarving throughout — waves leading up the staircase; flowers, vines, and sheaves of wheat on the mantels — the work of famous architect and woodcarver Samuel McIntire and his assistants. When admiring the staircase, notice the small piece of ivory inlaid in the newel post; that means the mortgage was paid off. You'll see the spacious parlor — scene of weddings, dances, and receptions — and the bedroom (indeed, the very bed) where one of the house's owners was murdered in a dispute over his will.

There are several other small buildings to explore on the institute property, but by this time your feet may need a rest. For a change of pace, go back into the museum building and watch the half-hour orientation slide show. The first segment concentrates on the history of the museum. The second segment covers the witchcraft trials and provides some intriguing facts (seventeenth-century prisoners were responsible for their own room and board bills) and speculation (some said a certain poisonous mold in the Puritans' bread caused a group of young girls to hallucinate and make the witchcraft accusations that led to all the trouble).

For deeper immersion in the witch hysteria, walk around the corner to the **Salem Witch Museum.** This is not a conventional museum but instead an intriguing multimedia presentation that takes place in the dark, with audience members standing in the center of a circular theater. "Do you believe in witches?" questions a disembodied voice. "Millions of your ancestors did." The voice goes on to describe the hysteria that afflicted some of the girls in seventeenth-century Salem. As the story unfolds, arrangements of mannequins are illuminated to complement the narration. Not only did prisoners have to pay for their food, but they also had to pay for the

Some said a certain poisonous mold in the Puritans' bread caused a group of young girls to hallucinate and make the witchcraft accusations that led to all the trouble.

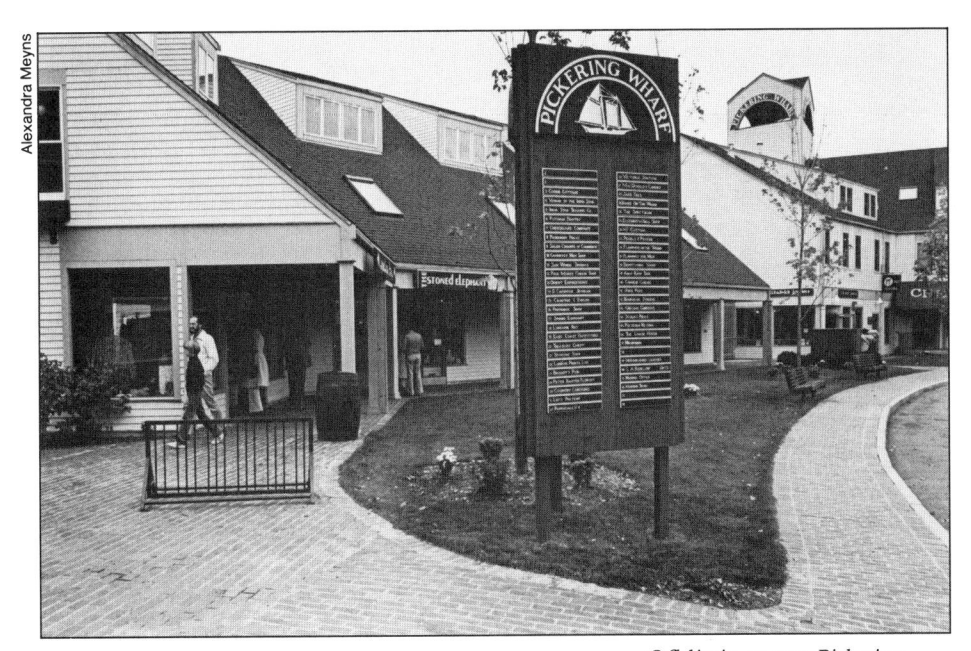

Off-limits to cars, Pickering Wharf is a pleasant place to stroll and shop year-round.

chains used to restrain them. You'll see accused witches caged like animals in tiny jail cells, atoning for crimes they never committed. And then, there's the scene atop Gallows Hill....

Move along next to **Pickering Wharf,** an upbeat, trendy complex of shops and restaurants edging the harbor. Pleasantly landscaped, with lots of benches and pretty lawns overlooking the water, much of Pickering Wharf is off-limits to cars, which makes it a good place to walk and window-shop. Special events scheduled throughout the year, from a waterfront festival in May to an October pumpkinfest, add to the cheerful atmosphere.

Just a short walk from Pickering Wharf is the **Salem Maritime National Historic Site,** where three wharves are all that remain of the more than fifty that once lined the harbor. The site testifies to Salem's stature as an important nineteenth-century port and to the importance of commercial shipping in the development of the American economy. You'll visit the Bonded Warehouse, the Scale House, and the Custom House, where merchants secured necessary permits and paid their customs taxes. At the West India Goods Store, where sugar, molasses, and tropical fruits from the Caribbean were sold alongside local products such as dried cod, nails, and fishhooks, you can purchase spices from the hundred plus wooden boxes that line one wall.

There are also three historic houses. The

A secret staircase, a closet with a false wall, and dark passageways await the visitor to the legendary House of Seven Gables.

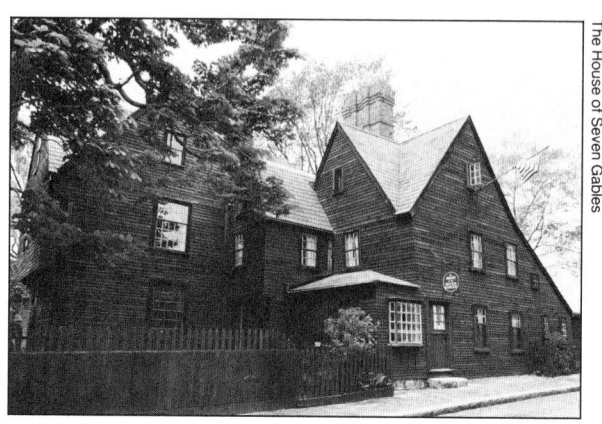

The House of Seven Gables

Hawkes House was designed by Salem's great architect, Samuel McIntire, and was used as a privateer prize warehouse during the American Revolution. The Narbonne–Hale House was built in the seventeenth century and was home to craftspeople and tradesmen. Our favorite is the Derby House, built in 1762 for ship owner Elias Hasket Derby, the city's most prominent merchant and probably the country's first millionaire.

The National Park Service conducts daily tours throughout the site. Pick up a schedule at the Central Wharf Warehouse Visitor Center on Derby Street as you enter the national historic site. All the programs begin in front of the Customs House. Examples of tours include a walk along Derby Wharf, with a discussion of Salem's shipping and trading days, and a forty-five-minute guided tour of the Derby House.

Continuing along Derby Street with the harbor to your right, you'll soon come to **Ye Olde Pepper Companie,** which calls itself the oldest candy company in the country, originating in 1806. This is the home of Black Jack Fudge, a molasses stick candy made from blackstrap molasses. Famous Salem Gibralters were invented here, too, by an early nineteenth-century Englishwoman whose family arrived destitute following a shipwreck. Neighbors, eager to lend a hand and aware of Mrs. Spencer's talents as a candy maker, donated a barrel of sugar, from which the industrious lady made the dainty lemon and peppermint–flavored rolls that were to become known as Salem Gibralters. She sold them more than a hundred years ago from a pail on the steps of the old First Church, and later from a wagon. Her business was bought from her son and heir by one Mr. Pepper, who began the company that continues today. You can still buy Gibralters at the Pepper

Companie, where you can also peer through large windows into the kitchen where candy makers heft paddles laden with white fondant as they prepare cream-center candies, fudges, jellies, and many other confections.

The entrance to the **House of Seven Gables,** immortalized in Nathaniel Hawthorne's novel of the same name, is just across the street from the candy company. The formal part of your visit is a forty-five-minute tour that begins with a brief slide show describing the house and Hawthorne's relationship to it. You'll discover that one of the author's ancestors was Judge John Hathorne, who presided over the 1692 witch trials. A witness at one of the trials is said to have placed a curse on the judge and his descendants, causing Nathaniel Hawthorne to remark of the past, "It lies upon the present like a giant's dead body."

You'll need to navigate steep staircases and dark passages in the house itself. In the kitchen, you'll see a seventeenth-century wine cabinet with hinges in the shape of an H, representing "heavenly" and "holy" and intended to keep the wine from going bad. Pass through the false back in the wood closet next to the fireplace and climb the secret, winding stairway that wraps around the massive cluster chimney. Bend low as you continue on through a dark passageway to the attic, descending next to the master bedroom, Phoebe's room in Hawthorne's novel.

The tour also includes a look at Hawthorne's birthplace, here on the same property. There's an inventory on the wall showing that Hawthorne's father's estate amounted to $338.60 at the time of his death, not enough to support his widow and three children, who soon sold this house and moved in with an uncle. In one of the upstairs bedrooms you'll see the bed where Nathaniel was born (it was used for births, deaths, and guests). The bedroom across the hall is painted Prussian blue, a color achieved by mixing crushed blueberries with sour milk. On the floor is a humane mouse catcher, used to capture but not kill the mouse, since the Puritans didn't believe in killing anything they didn't intend to eat. It even has a little wheel to give the creature exercise until it was released.

You'll want to allow time to stroll through the gardens, overlooking the harbor. Patterned after seventeenth-century Jacobean gardens, the flower beds contain more than fifty types of perennials,

In one of the upstairs bedrooms you'll see the bed where Nathaniel was born (it was used for births, deaths, and guests).

just as many flowering trees and shrubs, and thirty to forty types of annuals and bulbs. While you're walking, you may want to duck into the counting house, "a place for keeping books and transacting the business of a merchant or trader." A taped message (push the inconspicuous button high to the left of the glass display front) describes the furnishings and functions associated with the building. It's fun to have lunch at a table in the garden, out in the sun overlooking the harbor, or in the protective shade of the wisteria arbor. The self-service coffee shop prepares chowder, crabmeat salad rolls, fruit salad, and a selection of sandwiches. If the weather is poor, you can take a seat on a reproduction settle at one of the booths in the indoor dining area.

ACCESS

SALEM. Follow Route 128 north to exit 25E. Follow Route 114 east to Route 107. Turn left on Route 107, then right on Route 1A and continue into the center of Salem.

SALEM TROLLEY. Directions: Main office at Pickering Wharf, 59 Wharf Street. Trolley stops throughout the city, as indicated by trolley stop signs. You can buy your ticket and board at any point. **Season:** April through October. November and December weekends only. **Admission:** Charged. **Telephone:** (617) 744-5463.

PEABODY MUSEUM OF SALEM. Directions: From Route 128, take exit 25E. Follow Route 114 east about 2½ miles, then exit right onto Route 107 north (Bridge Street). Go right onto St. Peter Street, opposite the Parker Brothers factory. Park in the municipal parking lot and walk to the museum, which is located at East India Square. **Season:** Year-round. **Admission:** Charged; senior discount. **Telephone:** (617) 745-9500. **Note:** Most of museum is handicapped accessible.

ESSEX INSTITUTE. Directions: Located at 132 Essex Street. **Season:** Museum open year-round; historic houses open from June through October. **Admission:** Charged; senior discount. **Telephone:** (617) 744-3390.

SALEM WITCH MUSEUM. Directions: Located at Washington Square North, just off Hawthorne Boulevard (Route 1A) and just opposite Salem Common. **Season:** Year-round. **Admission:** Charged; senior discount. **Telephone:** (617) 744-1692.

PICKERING WHARF. Directions: Follow Route 1A to Derby Street. Turn left. Pickering Wharf is on the corner of Derby and Congress streets. **Season:** Year-round. **Admission:** Free. **Telephone:** (617) 745-9540.

SALEM MARITIME NATIONAL HISTORIC SITE. Directions: Sites are located along Derby Street on Salem

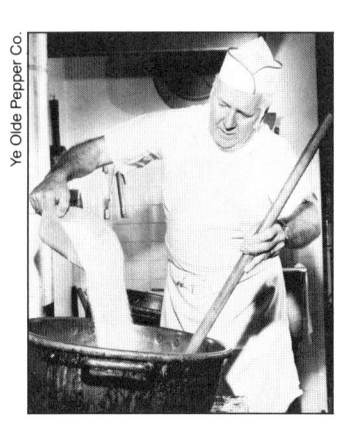

Ye Olde Pepper Companie candy makers has been a Salem favorite since 1806.

harbor. **Season:** Year-round; reduced tour schedule in the winter and spring. **Admission:** Free. **Telephone:** (617) 744-4323.

YE OLDE PEPPER COMPANIE. Directions: Located at 122 Derby Street on the waterfront. **Season:** Year-round. **Admission:** Free. **Telephone:** (617) 745-2744.

HOUSE OF SEVEN GABLES. Directions: Follow Derby Street east (the harbor to your right). Turn right on Turner Street opposite Ye Olde Pepper Companie and follow signs to house. (Parking is on Derby Street.) **Season:** Year-round; closed last 2 weeks in January. Garden coffee shop open May through October. **Admission:** Charged. **Telephone:** (617) 744-0991.

For further information or restaurant and lodging suggestions, contact the Salem Chamber of Commerce, Old Town Hall, 32 Derby Square, Salem, MA 01970. Telephone: (617) 744-0004.

Rockport

Spend a day, a week, or a month exploring a seaside artists' colony perched on the eastern tip of Cape Ann. Like most Massachusetts coastal towns, Rockport began as a fishing village. But in the early 1800s, Cape Ann's huge reserves of granite paved the way for a new industry. Craterlike quarries were dug, massive stone breakwaters were constructed, and quiet coves suddenly metamorphosed into busy shipping ports. The sleepy fishing village grew into a thriving terminal, exporting granite all over the United States and even to South America. The name Rockport, first used in the 1800s, testifies to the influence of the granite industry.

When advances in the use of cement and a shortage of skilled laborers led to the demise of the industry, Rockport quickly forged a new image, capitalizing this time on its natural beauty. Artists and writers began to cluster on Cape Ann in the mid-1800s, when itinerant painters traveled door to door, hoping to be hired to paint family portraits. The town's first studio was opened by the industrious Gilbert Tucker Margeson, who also ran a store and a telegraph agency and served as the local tax collector. By the 1920s Rockport had achieved a reputation as an artists' colony.

Today Rockport proudly reflects its past traditions. The quarries are no longer active, but the huge pits and heaps of stone slabs are a dramatic reminder

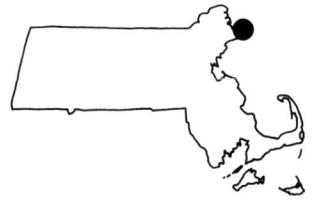

Artists and writers began to cluster on Cape Ann in the mid-1800s, when itinerant painters traveled door to door, hoping to be hired to paint family portraits.

of an industrial past. Art galleries and specialty shops line the downtown streets, occupying old wooden buildings that once housed fishing-related businesses, including a cooperage, a cod-liver oil works, and a net-making loft. You'll find studios, art supply stores, and frameries sprinkled along the wharves and streets, tucked between a mélange of elegant and quaint shops and restaurants. Virtually everything is within walking distance of everything else, and you have convenient access to the entire downtown area thanks to a park-and-ride shuttle service that spares you driving hassles during peak tourist season.

Wherever you wander in warm weather, you'll see painters at their easels. And wherever you ramble in town, you'll come across their work, even at the firehouse, the police station, and the town hall. Various painting workshops, lasting one or several days, provide you the chance to make your Rockport experience more than a casual visit.

The town also reflects its past in quite another way. If you enjoy a glass of wine or a cocktail with dinner, be sure to bring along your own provisions. There are no liquor stores in Rockport. Restaurants provide mixers, wineglasses, and the like, but they are prohibited from selling alcoholic beverages. This tradition dates back more than 130 years to the day when one Hannah Jumper, convinced of the evils of liquor, organized and led the "Women's Raid of 1856." Unfurling temperance banners and armed with hatchets, Hannah and her followers spent six hours bashing apart every keg of booze in the thirteen grog shops in town. Their work completed, they gathered in Dock Square at the foot of Bearskin Neck to congratulate themselves before heading home. To this day, Rockport remains a dry town. (If you want to see the very hatchets the women used, stop in at the **Sandy Bay Historical Society,** which also houses local artifacts relating to the fishing and granite industries.)

Bearskin Neck, a spit of land jutting out into the picture-perfect harbor, got its name in the early eighteenth century when Ebenezer Babson killed a bear there, skinned it, and stretched the pelt on the rocks to dry. Today lobster pounds and stores like The Pewter Shop, Mr. Bagman, and The Bearskin Neck Country Store line the streets, alleyways, and wharves. Here too you'll find Motif #1, the red fishing shack believed to be the most painted scene in America. (Actually, it's a reproduction; the original perished in the blizzard of 1978.)

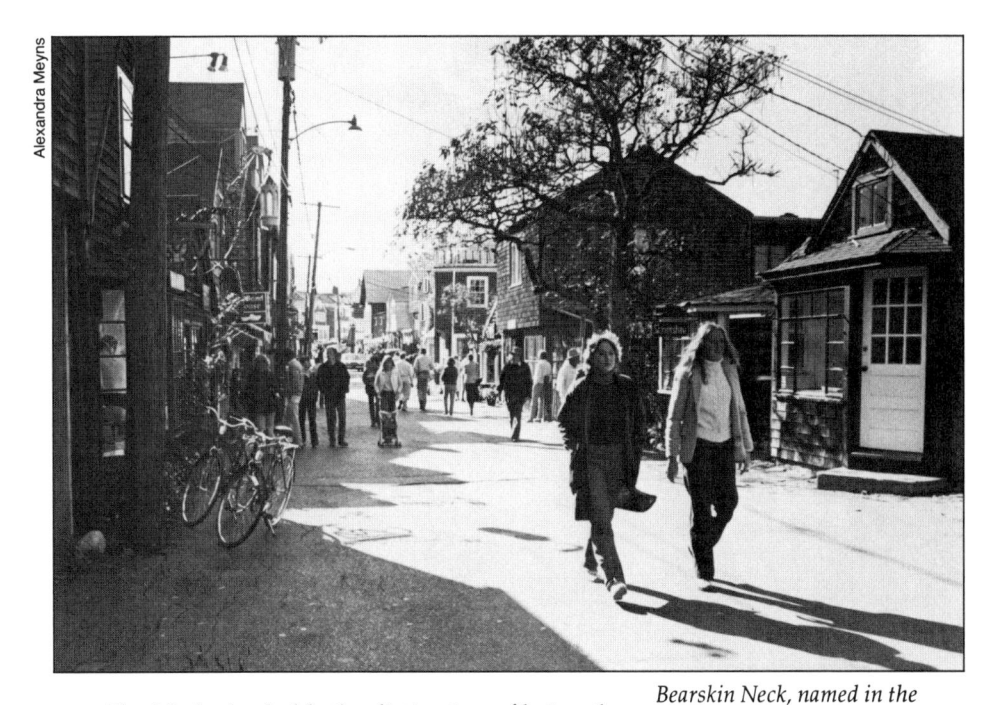

Bearskin Neck, named in the 1800s when a hunter stretched a bear pelt there to dry, is today the site of numerous shops and eateries.

The Neck also holds the distinction of being the home of the only mid-nineteenth-century producer of isinglass in the United States. In 1822 an enterprising fellow named William Hall started buying up fish bladders for pennies a pound. Using hand rollers, he flattened them into thin, clear sheets of gelatinous isinglass, a substance then used as a clarifying agent for wine and beer and an ingredient in adhesives and mock pearls.

Traffic in downtown Rockport can be a nightmare during the summer months. It's not simply that the town is thick with visitors, but there are lovely views of the sea wherever you look. People don't just drive through town; they linger. Parking is very limited on the narrow streets, further adding to the problem. Many visitors find it's best to ditch the car at the outlying parking lot and use the shuttle bus service included in the parking fee.

To get a feel for what's going on, begin your visit with a stop at the **Rockport Art Association** on Main Street. A bulletin board out front is chock-full of notices announcing lectures, plays, flea markets, church suppers, and just about anything else that's happening. The association was founded in 1921 and is housed in a two-hundred-year-old building that formerly served as a stop on the Rockport–Salem stagecoach line. Today it welcomes more than fifty thousand visitors a year. They come to admire the

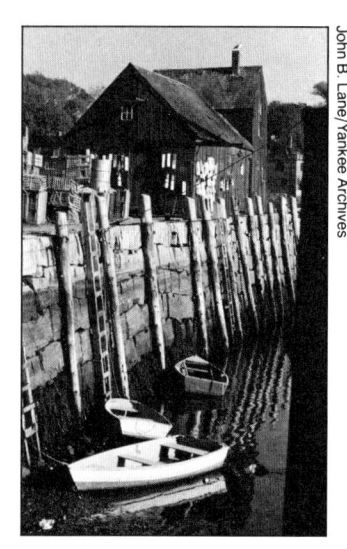

"Motif #1," the red fishing shack said to be the most painted scene in America, is actually a reproduction of the original, which was destroyed in a 1978 blizzard.

John B. Lane/Yankee Archives

paintings, drawings, sculpture, and photographs on exhibit and to purchase works by member artists.

The association hosts a lively schedule of events year-round, and visitors are welcome to participate. Portrait sketch groups and live model drawing groups meet several times a week (day and evening), and visitors can attend on a drop-in basis. Association member demonstrations are held each Tuesday and Thursday evening throughout the summer and early fall; subjects include self-portrait, mixed-media collage, seascape, figure composition, and others. You need only appear at the appointed hour.

A series of three-day intensive summer workshops in oil, watercolor, and mixed media also are offered for both beginners and experienced painters. These start with a wine and cheese get-together Sunday evening, continue with classes all day Monday and Tuesday and half a day Wednesday, and include evening lectures and demonstrations. An outdoor painting class is offered for those visiting briefly (even for just a day) who would like to go painting with a local artist. And the association sponsors frequent lectures and slide shows by area artists, writers, and art historians.

Rockport is also the home of the **Rockport Chamber Music Festival,** which features world-famous ensembles such as the Manhattan String Quartet, the Empire Trio, the Philadelphia-based Jubal Trio, and An die Musik. Launched six years ago by two New Yorkers, soprano Lila Deis (who has performed at Carnegie Hall and Lincoln Center) and composer/pianist David Alpher (founder of the New York Bach Ensemble), the festival runs for three weeks each June. Performances are held at the Rockport Art Association, which makes an ideal setting with its rafters, skylights, and walls lined with seascapes and country scenes. Just over two hundred people can fit into the folding chairs that are arranged in a semicircle in front of the small stage, providing the sense of intimacy appropriately associated with chamber music. During intermission, audience members enjoy refreshments and the opportunity to mingle with the performers.

Thanks to the direction of Deis and Alpher, imaginative programming has become a hallmark of the festival. The music offered in a typical season ranges from sixteenth century to twentieth, originating in places throughout Europe and the United States. Strings, brass, winds, keyboard, and voice are represented in forms that include fanfares, canzoni, songs, cantatas, and sonatas. Two visiting ensembles perform each week, separately on Thursday and Friday evenings, together on Saturday evenings and Sunday afternoons.

Another pleasant way to pass an evening is to take in a show at the **Little Art Cinema**. The auditorium is on the second floor of an old wood-frame meeting hall in downtown Rockport. It is the cleanest movie theater we've ever had the pleasure of visiting (nothing sticky about it!) and the only one we've ever encountered decorated with paper Tiffany-style lamp shades. The program changes at least twice a week, so it seems there's always something fresh to see. The fare includes a heavy dose of foreign films and classics.

During the day, you'll want to explore the many beaches, coves, quarries, and acres of woods. The **Rockport Conservation Commission** sponsors guided nature walks each weekend from late spring to early fall. Check the Art Association bulletin board for details. Your guide will fill you in on the history and ecology of the area and will help you identify the flora and fauna. Keep an eye out for the scarlet tanagers that make their home in the interior of Cape Ann, as well as for the delicate wild orchids that thrive in damp spots. Wild blueberries also proliferate here, and you might want to return on your own later to fill up a bucket to take home. If you are a bird-watcher, you may want to make a fall pilgrimage out to **Andrews Point** to watch the spectacle of the annual autumn sea bird migration, when guillemots, dovekies, and even puffins head south for the winter in a nonstop panorama.

Front Beach and **Back Beach** are located within a five-minute walk of each other right on the edge of the downtown shopping area. Front Beach is a good place to stretch out in the sun or just enjoy the view of Sandy Bay and the curve of Bearskin Neck beyond. Back Beach is rocky but well protected. It affords a fine view of the bay and of Straitsmouth Light. There's an old-fashioned bandstand right across the street where band concerts are held each Sunday evening during the summer. (From the center of Rockport, follow Main Street which becomes Beach Street. Both beaches will be on your right.)

Just across the street from Front Beach, you'll see a modest green-and-white clapboard stand with a sign reading **"No-Key."** Go inside and you'll feel as though you've stepped back into the 1950s. Take a seat at the counter or wait for a space at one of the half dozen plastic-covered tables and enjoy a frappe, a steamed hot dog, or maybe a plate of fried clams. If

Make a fall pilgrimage out to Andrews Point to watch guillemots, dovekies, and even puffins head south for the winter.

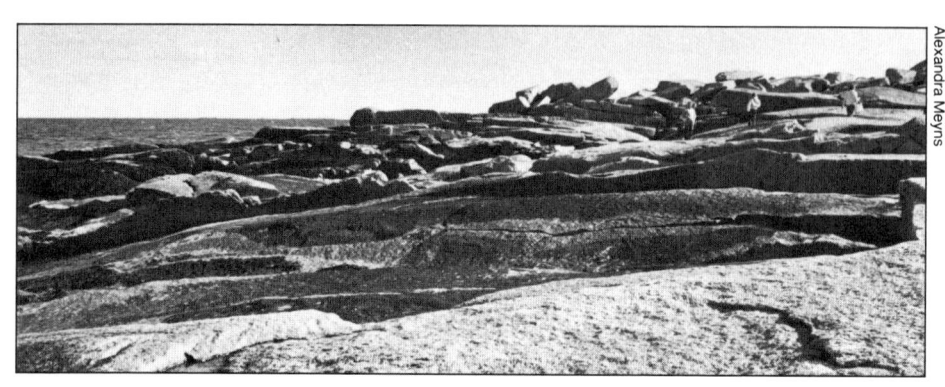

Once a large granite quarry, Halibut Point Reservation today "must be one of the most spectacular picnic spots in New England."

No-Key is too crowded for your liking, get your order to go and carry it outside to adjacent **Millbrook Meadow,** a gracious public park complete with swings, benches, and even its own waterfall and millpond. It provides the perfect in-town picnic spot, a quiet oasis even at the height of summer.

If you want to get out on the water, you can opt for a whale watch aboard **Captain Ted's Rockport Whale Watching,** signing on for a half-day trip to see the huge animals perform. For those who prefer a tamer form of seagoing, Captain Ted also offers daily one-hour island excursions, which give you close-ups of Straitsmouth, Milk, and Thatcher islands (the last named for Anthony Thatcher and his wife, who survived a tragic shipwreck near here in 1635, in which their four children and twenty-one other people perished). For the fisherman, Captain Ted provides five-hour party boat trips. He'll supply the bait and tackle (or you can bring your own), and you'll angle for cod, haddock, and pollock. If you prefer to do your fishing from terra firma, take a short ride out to **Granite Pier Wharf** (also accessible by trolley), a long stone jetty where hand-line fishing is permitted. On a summer day, this is also a good vantage point for watching the sailboat races that float across Sandy Bay.

For a close-up of one of the large quarries, continue south past Granite Pier Wharf to **Halibut Point Reservation**. Owned and maintained by the Trustees of Reservations, the point includes an enormous quarry, now filled with water. A well-maintained broad dirt trail circles the brim of the pit, offering views of the spring-fed quarry with its flat granite sides and, in the distance, the open sea — all in the same vista. If you are willing to contend with more difficult footing, you can make your way along the rough, stony paths that lead toward the ocean. You'll see a huge slag heap of scrap granite towering high above the flat shelves of rock that stretch out into the bay where the ocean bangs unmercifully. We can't help thinking this must be one of the most spectacular picnic spots in New England, no matter that the competition be fierce! By the way, you can get to Halibut Point and back into the center of town via the trolley.

It would be a mistake to stereotype Rockport exclusively as a summer destination. Most of the shops and many of the inns and restaurants stay open through the Christmas holidays, and a good number offer attractive off-season rates, particularly after Columbus Day. There are special weekend events throughout December, including the tree-lighting ceremony, the ice sculpture exhibition, and a forty-year tradition, the **Annual Christmas Pageant** (always the Saturday before Christmas). A torchlit reenactment of the Nativity, the outdoor procession complete with live animals, wends its way through downtown, while a voice tells the Christmas story over a loudspeaker.

There are church fairs and festivals throughout the month, and musical performances — including a cappella choirs, brass quartets, Finnish singers, Scandinavian dancers, school groups, and bell ringers — are held each weekend. For a real treat Rockport-style, reserve a place at the **Yuletide Smorgasbord,** held at the Peg Leg Restaurant from noon to 7 P.M. on the day of the pageant. A calendar of events for **Christmas in Rockport** is available from the Cape Ann Chamber of Commerce.

Most of the shops and many of the inns and restaurants stay open through the Christmas holidays, and a good number offer attractive off-season rates.

ACCESS

ROCKPORT. Follow Route 128 north to the Gloucester rotary. Take the second exit off the rotary, following signs to Rockport, a distance of about 4 miles. You will pass a pay parking lot on your left before entering town. Fee entitles you to use shuttle bus into town, a good idea during peak season, when parking is often a problem. Shuttle runs from Memorial Day through Labor Day.

SANDY BAY HISTORICAL SOCIETY. Directions: Located at 40 King Street. **Season:** July 1 through Labor Day and weekends in September. **Admission:** Donation requested. **Telephone:** (617) 546-9533.

ROCKPORT ART ASSOCIATION. Directions: Located at 12 Main Street in the center of Rockport. **Season:** Year-round. **Admission:** Free; fees charged for programs. **Telephone:** (617) 546-6604.

ROCKPORT CHAMBER MUSIC FESTIVAL. Directions: Performances are held at the Rockport Art Association on Main Street. **Season:** June. **Admission:** Charged. **Telephone:** (617) 546-6604.

LITTLE ART CINEMA. Directions: Located at 18 Broadway in downtown Rockport. **Season:** Mid-June through Labor Day. **Admission:** Charged. **Telephone:** (617) 546-2548.

ROCKPORT CONSERVATION COMMISSION WALKS. Directions: Walks depart from different points. Call the Cape Ann Chamber of Commerce for particulars. **Season:** May through October. **Admission:** Free. Donations requested. **Telephone:** (617) 283-1601.

ANDREWS POINT. Directions: Follow Route 127 in the direction of Gloucester. Turn right on Phillips Avenue, about 2 miles out of downtown Rockport. Continue to end of road. **Season:** Year-round. **Admission:** Free. **Telephone:** None.

MILLBROOK. Directions: Located at 16 Beach Street, opposite Front Beach. **Season:** Year-round. **Admission:** Free. **Telephone:** (617) 546-9656.

CAPTAIN TED'S ROCKPORT WHALE WATCHING. Directions: Trips depart from Tuna Wharf in downtown Rockport. **Season:** May through September. **Admission:** Charged. **Telephone:** (617) 546-2889.

GRANITE PIER WHARF. Directions: Traveling south on Route 127 (Granite Street), turn right on Wharf Road, which leads to the pier. **Season:** Year-round. **Admission:** Parking fee (summer only). **Telephone:** None.

HALIBUT POINT RESERVATION. Directions: Follow Route 127 (Granite Street) south toward Gloucester. Turn right onto Gott Street, following signs to reservation parking area. **Season:** Year-round. **Admission:** Parking fee. **Telephone:** (617) 283-1601.

CHRISTMAS IN ROCKPORT. Directions: Activities are located throughout town. Contact the Cape Ann Chamber of Commerce for a calendar of events. **Season:** December. **Admission:** Free to most events. **Note:** For reservations for the Yuletide Smorgasbord, call the Peg Leg Restaurant at (617) 546-3038.

For further information or restaurant and lodging suggestions, contact the Cape Ann Chamber of Commerce, 33 Commercial Street, Gloucester, MA 01930. Telephone: (617) 283-1601.

Sheffield

In marked contrast to its neighbors to the north, Great Barrington and Stockbridge, Sheffield is a serene, pastoral town. As one local happily explained, "There's no large, central hotel here, so we don't get the great influx of visitors that gather elsewhere in the southern Berkshires." Sheffield has the scenery without the traffic and crowds. The town also offers outdoor activities to suit every taste and fitness level. Whether you favor a walk through an unspoiled meadow, a steep hill climb, or a day of paddling on a gentle river, you'll find Sheffield can deliver handsomely. It is a fine daytrip destination, and if you are planning a visit to one of its well-known neighbors, you'll find it a pleasant respite from the more frenetic pace they offer.

The town of Sheffield itself is an antiquer's paradise, with at least ten shops to explore right along Route 7 and another half dozen just minutes away in Ashley Falls. As you wander through their nooks and crannies, you'll feel as though you've returned to your grandparents' home. Most of the shops are open year-round. You can get a map showing the locations of the shops and describing the specialties of each by writing to the Berkshire County Office of Tourism.

To see the dealers at work buying their stock and to try your own luck at securing a find in a competitive atmosphere, attend an auction at **Bradford Galleries, Ltd.**, where sales are held once each month except March and April. The antiques put up for bid here come mostly from area homes and estate sales. Auctioneer William Bradford has been in the business for over twenty years, and he knows how to keep sales moving. Bradford disposes of about seventy lots per hour, which means the pace is brisk and the buyer best be prepared.

That's possible, though, because all the sales are cataloged and there is always at least a three-day preview period during which potential buyers are welcome to scrutinize the pieces close up. A catalog from a recent sale listed 379 lots of miscellaneous antiques and 51 lots of books. The description of each lot is accompanied by an estimate of the low and high price each piece is likely to fetch. Here's a sample listing: "5 fine cut glass tumblers diamond and fan pattern, 4" ht. 200/300."

At the front of each catalog is a timetable indicating the approximate time of day when each category will go up for sale. If you're specifically inter-

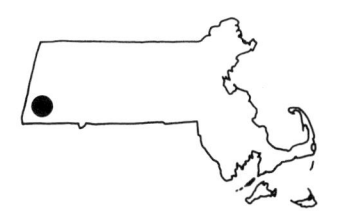

The town of Sheffield itself is an antiquer's paradise.

ested in cut glass, for example, you'll know that those pieces are likely to come up between 1:30 and 1:45 P.M. Of course, that's not exact, and you should get there early, but it does mean that you don't have to arrive when the sale starts at 11 A.M. in order to bid on the vase that caught your eye at the preview. All sales are held during the day on the weekend, under a tent in warm weather and indoors in cold. Two hundred to three hundred people attend each sale. Hot dogs and sandwiches are available.

The gallery also runs substantial prepriced tag sales four or five times a year. This is when you can pick up modern furnishings and odds and ends that wouldn't attract much attention at auction. Instead of putting together miscellaneous small items to form a single box lot at auction as some auctioneers do, the Bradfords save the less important items for their tag sales.

For a different type of shopping, stop in at **Sheffield Pottery,** where you can purchase pottery made on the premises from clay dug there. Sheffield Pottery features a distinctive line of brown and white ware, a design rooted in folk art produced by European peasants over a thousand years ago. In addition to first-quality pieces, the store sells seconds at inexpensive prices. Housed in a rambling red barn, the shop is filled with shelves of mugs, plates, pitchers, bean pots, bowls, creamers, and pie plates in lots of attractive designs. Clay, glazes, and tools and equipment for home potters are also available.

The quiet and beauty of the countryside are no better experienced than by paddling a canoe along the gentle stretch of the Housatonic River that drifts past Sheffield.

The quiet and beauty of the countryside are no better experienced than by paddling a canoe along the gentle stretch of the Housatonic River that drifts past Sheffield. The people at **Pedal and Paddle** will provide everything you need for a leisurely three-and-a-half-hour paddling foray down the river, where they will meet you with your car. This is a tranquil stretch of water, very easy to navigate, yet you'll feel a million miles removed from civilization. You won't see any houses along the way, but you may well catch sight of egrets, beavers, and perhaps an opossum or deer. The property on either side of the river, stretching ten yards back, belongs to the state, so you are free to break for a picnic or a swim or just to rest along the way. If you plan to tour the Berkshires by river on a weekend, it's best to call in advance to reserve a canoe.

Pedal and Paddle also rents bicycles. No regular bikes these, but eighteen-speed models that just about erase hills. All you have to do is get the hang of all that shifting.

Bartholomew's Cobble nature sanctuary in Ashley Falls boasts 277 beautiful acres.

Speaking of picnics, Pedal and Paddle will supply a lunch for you to take along — anything from sandwiches to a full gourmet meal. Pedal and Paddle's proprietor doubles as the proprietor of the local package store, so if you want a bottle of fine wine or some imported beer included, just let him know. The picnics are prepared by **Mary's Place,** a small restaurant located in the back half of the package store building. Chutney chicken salad and Mediterranean salad are favorite picnic items, but Mary is also willing to assemble a feast of cold poached lobster, cold soup, fruit, and pâté. She can supply all the cutlery and tableware, too, right down to the wineglasses. Simple lunches are available on the spot, while more ambitious meals require a day's notice.

Even if you don't need a picnic, you might want to have lunch in this pleasant café. Crisp print curtains frame the windows, and bentwood chairs and small wooden tables, each decorated with a bouquet of dried flowers, provide the seating. The menu changes daily but usually includes a few specialties such as herbed chicken salad with walnuts or spinach and warm chèvre salad with poached pears and raspberry dressing, along with fresh breads, soups, and salads.

If you'd like to put together your own impromptu box lunch, try **The Corn Crib,** nestled beneath a huge weeping willow tree just north of town. This large indoor/outdoor farm stand sells all sorts of fresh local produce along with freshly baked bread and homemade cookies and fruit pies. The stand also stocks a good selection of cheeses, including some tasty local Cheddars, and Vermont honey, syrup, jams, and jellies.

The competition is fierce, but it's difficult to imagine there can be a more beautiful place in western Massachusetts to dine alfresco than **Bartholomew's Cobble,** a 277-acre nature sanctuary belonging to the nonprofit Trustees of Reservations, the largest private owner of conservation land in the state. Cobbles are rocky outcrops formed as long ago as fifty million years. More than eight hundred species of plants grow here, including forty-four varieties of ferns and many rare wildflowers. The terrain varies from a natural rock garden to a forest of hardwood and coniferous trees to meadows and pastureland. A network of trails, some quite steep, winds through the preserve and to the top of Hurlburt's Hill, which offers splendid views of the Housatonic Valley.

The **Ledges Interpretive Trail,** a half-mile loop, winds along the banks of the Housatonic River. At the tiny natural history museum on the property you can purchase a guide booklet that identifies plant life and geological features at the twenty numbered posts situated along the trail. The first half of the route is fairly steep in spots, with rough stairs to navigate. The second half is easy walking, largely flat and grassy underfoot. If you prefer to avoid the early part, just walk the trail backward, beginning at the end and continuing to perhaps post 12 before retracing your steps for the return. Allow about forty-five minutes to travel the trail, unless of course you bring along a picnic to spread out in a perfect meadow ablaze with pink, yellow, and blue wildflowers.

Within half a mile of the Cobble, you can visit the **Colonel Ashley House,** which is also a property of the Trustees of Reservations. Built in 1735 by John Ashley, the commanding beige clapboard house, oldest dwelling in Berkshire County, sits on a quiet

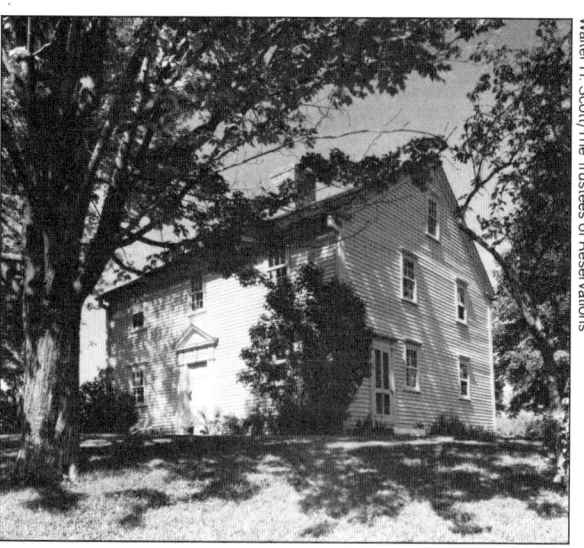

The Colonel Ashley House, built in 1735 by John Ashley, is the oldest dwelling in Berkshire County.

74 / MASSACHUSETTS

country road amidst a backdrop of corn fields and rolling hills. A man of many talents, Ashley was a pioneer, legislator, judge, and lawyer, as well as an officer in the French and Indian War. A loyal patriot, he also furnished iron and supplies for the American Revolution. It is believed that a list of fourteen resolutions against British tyranny (which came to be called the Sheffield Declaration of Independence because of its similarity to the famous Declaration of Independence drafted in Philadelphia three and a half years later) was drafted here in Ashley's study.

Another indication of Ashley's importance is the 1781 incident regarding one of his slaves, Mum Bett. She fled from this house and eventually went to court and successfully sued for her own freedom. By dropping his privilege of appeal, Colonel Ashley became the first man in Massachusetts to recognize abolition as provided for in the new state constitution. You'll learn more about him as you take a guided tour through his home, which contains eighteenth- and nineteenth-century furnishings, along with a tool collection and unusual pottery.

A man of many talents, Ashley was a pioneer, legislator, judge, and lawyer, as well as an officer in the French and Indian War.

ACCESS

SHEFFIELD. Follow I-90, Massachusetts Turnpike, to exit 1. Take Route 41 south to Route 7. Continue south on Route 7 into Sheffield.

BRADFORD GALLERIES, LTD. Directions: Located on Route 7 in Sheffield. **Season:** Year-round; usually no auctions in March and April. **Admission:** Free. **Telephone:** (413) 229-6667.

SHEFFIELD POTTERY. Directions: Located on Route 7 in Sheffield just north of the center of town. **Season:** Year-round. **Admission:** Free. **Telephone:** (413) 229-7700.

PEDAL AND PADDLE. Directions: Located in the Sheffield Package Store on Route 7 in the center of town. **Season:** Late March through late October. **Admission:** Free. **Telephone:** (413) 229-3033.

MARY'S PLACE. Directions: Located in the rear of the Sheffield Package Store on Route 7. **Season:** April through January. **Admission:** Free. **Telephone:** (413) 229-8784.

THE CORN CRIB. Directions: Located on Route 7, north of the center of town. **Season:** Year-round. **Admission:** Free. **Telephone:** None.

BARTHOLOMEW'S COBBLE. Directions: From Sheffield center follow Route 7 south 1 mile. Turn right on Route 7A and follow signs. **Season:** Mid-April through mid-October. **Admission:** Charged. **Telephone:** (413) 298-3239.

COLONEL ASHLEY HOUSE. Directions: From Sheffield center, follow Route 7 south 1 mile. Turn right on Route 7A and follow signs. **Season:** June through October; closed some weekends, call ahead. **Admission:** Charged. **Telephone:** (413) 298-3239.

For a listing of antique shops in Sheffield and the surrounding area, or for restaurant and lodging suggestions, contact the Southern Berkshire Chamber of Commerce, 362 Main Street, P.O. Box 510, Great Barrington, MA 01230. Telephone: (413) 528-1510.

Williamstown and North Adams

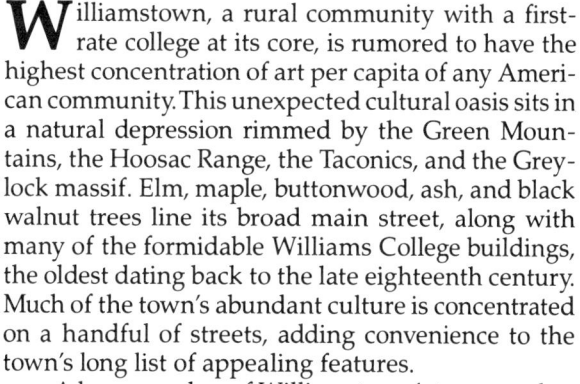

Williamstown, a rural community with a first-rate college at its core, is rumored to have the highest concentration of art per capita of any American community. This unexpected cultural oasis sits in a natural depression rimmed by the Green Mountains, the Hoosac Range, the Taconics, and the Greylock massif. Elm, maple, buttonwood, ash, and black walnut trees line its broad main street, along with many of the formidable Williams College buildings, the oldest dating back to the late eighteenth century. Much of the town's abundant culture is concentrated on a handful of streets, adding convenience to the town's long list of appealing features.

A large number of Williamstown's treasures belong to the **Sterling and Francine Clark Art Institute,** with its important collection of French nineteenth-century paintings. Here you'll find many examples of Renoir's work, along with works of other famous impressionists including Monet, Degas, Pissarro, and Sisley. Particularly noteworthy among the paintings by older masters is the rare panel painting by Piero della Francesca, *Virgin and Child Enthroned with Four Angels.* Gainsborough, Turner, and Goya are represented in the small collection of English and Spanish paintings. There are also major works by American artists Homer, Sargent, Cassatt, and Remington.

That's just the beginning. The Institute also has prints and drawings from the fifteenth to early twentieth century, by such masters as Rembrandt, Daumier, Toulouse-Lautrec, Gauguin, and Dürer. The sculpture collection includes bronzes by Rodin, Renoir, and Degas. Examples of seventeenth- and eighteenth-century English silver predominate in the decorative arts department, which also has fine

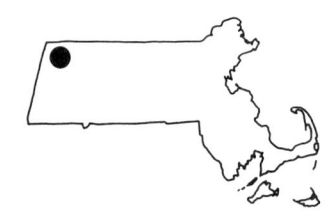

Williamstown, a rural community with a first-rate college at its core, is rumored to have the highest concentration of art per capita of any American community.

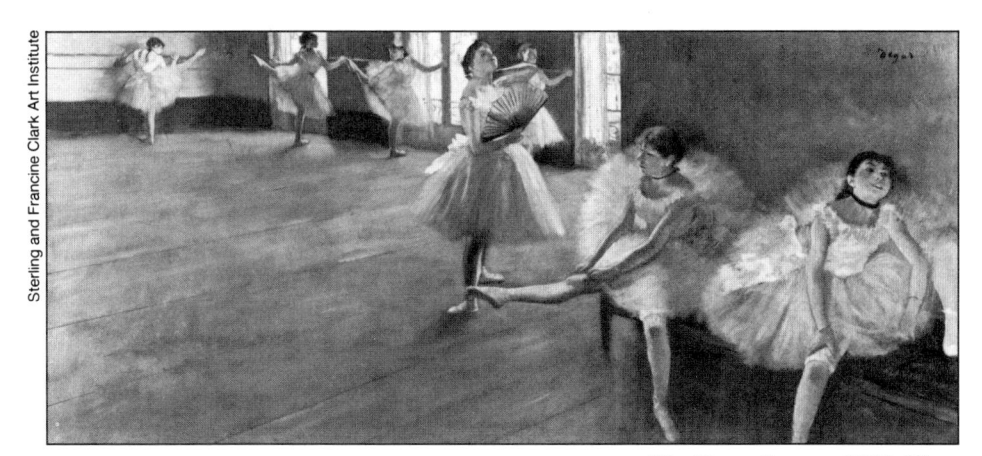

The Dance Lesson (1883–85), by Edgar Degas, is one of many treasures exhibited at Williamstown's Clark Art Institute.

examples of American, French, and Dutch craftsmanship, spanning more than three centuries. Other collections include eighteenth- and nineteenth-century porcelain from the Meissen, Chantilly, and Sèvres factories; early American glass; and French and American furniture. The institute is a sizable museum, and you will want to take your time wandering through the galleries, perhaps taking a break to enjoy lunch at the outdoor café in good weather.

In contrast to the Clark Institute, the **Williams College Museum of Art,** which has a permanent collection of about ten thousand pieces, focuses on twentieth-century American and South Asian art. With shiny hardwood floors, high-ceilinged galleries with huge skylights, and sophisticated exhibit spaces, the museum (which recently underwent a six-year, $8 million architectural renovation program) is an adaptable setting and the ideal showcase for major traveling shows. Simultaneously on display recently were "Die Revision der Modern" (a visiting exhibition focusing on postmodern architecture), a faculty show, and selections from the museum's permanent collection, which encompasses pieces as diverse as a late sixteenth-century Flemish portrait of the Archduchess Isabella Clara Eugenia and a huge twentieth-century Andy Warhol acrylic and silkscreen on canvas self-portrait. You are also likely to see works representative of the museum's extensive collection of paintings by Maurice and Charles Prendergast. Films and lectures by artists and art professors are offered on Wednesdays and Saturdays.

Performing arts flourish alongside fine arts in Williamstown. Founded in 1955, the **Williamstown Theatre Festival** stages professional performances of theater classics at the Williams College Adams

Memorial Theatre. Famous actors such as Christopher Reeve, Joanne Woodward, and Richard Chamberlain return again and again to perform in time-proven works by playwrights such as Tennessee Williams and Anton Chekhov. In addition to the main stage plays, small-scale Equity productions are offered by "The Other Stage," a branch of the festival emphasizing new works that performs in a different section of the same building. Indicative of the caliber of festival productions is the fact that ten of thirteen recent premières of new plays have gone on to commercial productions in New York and other cities. The festival also runs a cabaret program.

If you like foreign and art films, check the schedule at the **Images Cinema,** where the fare varies from recent releases to imports to cult films popular with the college crowd. The program changes every few days. A typical month's listing included *My Sweet Little Village,* a Czech film portrait of a small Czechoslovakian village; *Therese,* a French production about the French Carmelite nun Therese Martin; and *Waiting for the Moon,* an American movie focusing on the relationship between Alice B. Toklas and Gertrude Stein, two of this century's most intriguing literary figures.

The **Erasmus Café** on Spring Street, which favors light "bistro-style" fare, seems just the right place to dine after visiting art museums. The Erasmus serves three meals a day and stays open until midnight from May through December, which also makes it an excellent place to stop in for a drink or a fabulous after-theater dessert, like a slab of white chocolate mousse cake or Raspberry Rhapsody (a two-layer chocolate cake filled with raspberry mousse and coated with a hard chocolate shell). Eat outdoors under a striped umbrella on the elevated terrace decorated with geranium-filled window boxes, or indoors at one of the small, elegantly appointed tables tucked into the space the café shares with **The College Bookstore**. A tiny semicircular wooden counter also seats six. The shelves of books, the abundant greenery, and the classical music that is often playing in the background make the café an easy place to relax.

For breakfast (served anytime) try a filled omelette, for lunch a cup of cool Scandinavian melon soup or a crock of smoked bluefish mousse with fresh bread. Or perhaps you'd fancy chicken and pasta salad, or ratatouille in a pocket. If the weather is chilly, warm up with mocha cappuccino; fine wines and imported beers are served as well. The

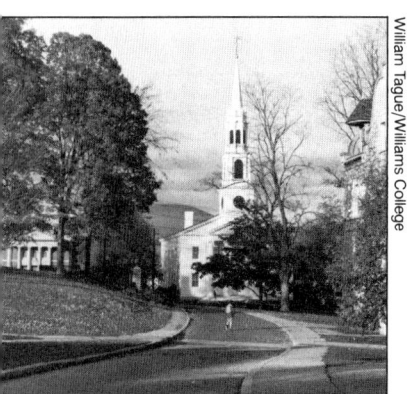

The cultural allure of Williamstown is, in part, thanks to the presence of Williams College, whose oldest buildings date back to the late 1700s.

café also can fix you up with a gourmet picnic to take along on your travels.

Confusing as this may seem, The College Bookstore is not really *the* college bookstore. If you would like to browse in the store that stocks the books required by students at Williams, head for the **Williams Bookstore,** on the same street as The College Bookstore. In addition to textbooks, you'll find clearly marked sections devoted to literature, poetry, music, philosophy, art, theater, dance, and other branches of the humanities. There's also an excellent selection of Penguin mysteries from which to choose.

From Williamstown, it's easy to make a sidetrip to nearby North Adams, home of **Western Gateway Heritage State Park**. The park consists of a complex of restored nineteenth-century wooden railroad buildings that open onto a cobblestone courtyard. A part of the Massachusetts Urban Heritage State Park Program — a national model in urban landscape design, historic preservation, and economic revitalization — the North Adams facility celebrates the city's proud industrial past, particularly its days as a railroad boomtown.

The heart of the park is the visitor center, with its long freight deck and working railroad crossing sign that lights up when real freight trains pass on a nearby track. Covered with old woodcuts, maps, newspaper clippings, train schedules, photographs, and related ephemera, a series of panels at the center relate the history of the Hoosac Valley. Isolated and dangerous in the 1700s, the area was cut off from the coast by steep and treacherous mountains and was constantly under threat of attack by the French and their Indian allies. In 1741 Fort Massachusetts was built at the future site of North Adams, but the Indians promptly burned it. The fort was rebuilt, and eventually the French and Indians withdrew, leaving the British to settle.

Because the acidic soil, rocks, and hills made farming difficult, many of the early settlers soon turned to lumbering, using waterpower from the Hoosac River to power their mills, of which there were a dozen (including gristmills) by the mid-1790s. North Adams evolved into a still more complex manufacturing town with the advent of the Industrial Revolution in the early 1800s, producing cotton and woolen cloth, boots and shoes, and printed and dyed textiles. Workers also forged iron, built machines, and made stone and wood products.

Geographic isolation continued to be a serious

In 1741 Fort Massachusetts was built at the future site of North Adams, but the Indians promptly burned it.

problem, particularly with the increased need to ship goods to market. Work on the Hoosac Tunnel, designed to connect North Adams to the eastern industrial cities and the seacoast by rail, began in 1851. The completion of the tunnel in 1875 marked one of the greatest engineering feats of the nineteenth century — the world's longest railroad tunnel. By 1900 more than a hundred trains a day passed through the tunnel.

You'll get a feel for the politics of the day and for the travails of the men who worked on the project as you approach a hall designed to simulate a tunnel and hear men chipping away with pickaxes, water dripping, and shovels scraping. You'll discover that the Hoosac Mountain rock seams held tons of water and that the miners often worked in downpour conditions, wearing heavy boots and raincoats and using oil lamps for illumination. Tape-recorded voices argue the economics of the project, reflecting a battle between New York and Boston for control of the inland markets. Take a seat on a barrel or box in front of a diorama of miners and listen to their accents, reflecting their ethnic diversity, as they "talk" about a blasting accident and wonder aloud, "You got any idea when we're going to break through to the western front?"

The visitor center also includes a small theater where you can watch old railroad films chronicling the days of steam, diesel, and electric locomotion. Free guided tours of the old railroad yard and the park buildings are offered throughout the day. Do call in advance to reserve space on the tours.

Need a snack to revive yourself? Take a look around the **North Adams General Store,** right in the park. Your nose will immediately discover that there's a bakery on the premises. Treat yourself to some shortbread cookies, gingersnaps, or a fresh cinnamon-raisin bun. There's also an adjoining ice cream parlor serving shakes, sundaes, and cones in flavors such as praline pecan, orange pineapple, and spumoni. The rest of the shop is filled with gift items that include kitchen gadgets, wicker pieces, candles, potpourri, soaps, and the like.

Two miles from the Western Gateway you can visit **Natural Bridge State Park,** developed around a huge white marble formation that forms a natural bridge and dates back about 500 million years. The site also boasts a huge quarry and a marble dam. A valued building material, the coarse-grained white marble from the bridge area was used for tombstones and for construction of the old Phoenix Hotel in North Adams. The first European to discover the natural bridge was a hunter who worked for Fort Massachusetts in the mid-1700s. As the hunter was returning to the fort with a deer one night, the animal slipped from his grasp and plunged into a chasm. When he returned by daylight with soldiers from the fort to help him retrieve the deer, they discovered the dramatic formation. As Nathaniel Hawthorne wrote in one of his American Notebooks after visiting the area in 1838, "The cave makes a fresh impression on me every time I visit it ... so deep, so irregular, so gloomy, so stern."

Another outdoor attraction worthy of attention is the ten-thousand-acre expanse known as **Mount Greylock State Reservation**. The area contains thirty-five miles of hiking trails, including a stretch of the Appalachian Trail, which runs from Maine to Georgia. An easy way to enjoy the pleasures of the reservation is to visit **Bascom Lodge** at the summit of Mount Greylock, the state's highest peak at 3,491 feet. Constructed by the Civilian Conservation Corps in the 1930s, the rustic stone-and-wood lodge can accommodate thirty guests in private and dormitory-style rooms. Linens are supplied, but you're advised to bring along extra blankets or a sleeping bag when the weather is cool. A sandwich bar is open all day, and hearty breakfasts and dinners are served family-style. You needn't be an overnight guest to eat at the lodge, but reservations are required.

Two Appalachian Mountain Club (AMC) naturalists stationed at the lodge offer information and suggestions for hikes, lead guided nature walks, and present evening programs on area history, geology, and plant and animal life. In addition, one- and two-day workshops are offered throughout the season, covering topics that range from bird watching to geology to photography. Write in advance for a schedule and more information about the lodge, its facilities, and its programs.

Because of its altitude, cool damp climate, and thick vegetation, Mount Greylock attracts several birds that never or rarely breed elsewhere in the state. These include the Bicknell's thrush, mourning warbler, blackpoll warbler, olive-sided flycatcher, red-breasted nuthatch, brown creeper, winter wren, olive-backed thrush, and golden-crowned kinglet. Three types of hawks — the accipiters, buteos, and falcons — can be seen flying over the mountain. Barred owls and great horned owls are frequent resi-

The Mount Greylock State Reservation contains thirty-five miles of hiking trails, including a stretch of the Appalachian Trail.

Having recently undergone an $8 million renovation, the Williams College Museum of Art provides a magnificent setting for both permanent and traveling exhibits.

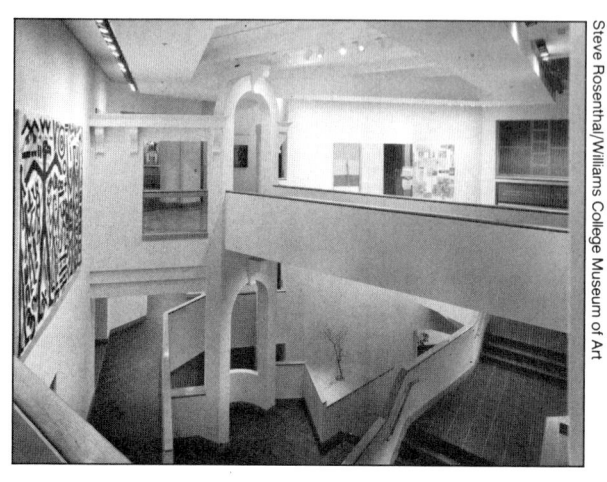

dents. The Massachusetts Department of Environmental Management prints a leaflet called "Birds of Mt. Greylock," which you can request by writing to the lodge.

ACCESS

WILLIAMSTOWN. Take I-91 to Route 2 west (Mohawk Trail) to Williamstown.

NORTH ADAMS. Take I-91 to Route 2 west (Mohawk Trail) to Route 8. Go south on Route 8 into North Adams.

STERLING AND FRANCINE CLARK ART INSTITUTE. Directions: Follow Route 2 (Main Street) west through Williamstown. Turn left onto South Street at the intersection with Route 7. Located at 225 South Street in Williamstown. **Season:** Year-round. **Admission:** Free. **Telephone:** (413) 458-9545. **Note:** Museum is handicapped accessible, and wheelchairs are available.

WILLIAMS COLLEGE MUSEUM OF ART. Directions: Located on Main Street (Route 2) in Williamstown. **Season:** Year-round. **Admission:** Free. **Telephone:** (413) 597-2429.

WILLIAMSTOWN THEATRE FESTIVAL. Directions: Performances held in the Adams Memorial Theatre on Main Street (Route 2) in Williamstown. **Season:** Late June through late August. **Admission:** Charged. **Telephone:** (413) 597-3400.

IMAGES CINEMA. Directions: Follow Route 2 (Main Street) west into the center of Williamstown. Turn left on Spring Street. Located at 50 Spring Street in Williamstown. **Season:** Year-round. **Admission:** Charged. **Telephone:** (413) 458-5612.

ERASMUS CAFÉ and THE COLLEGE BOOKSTORE. Directions: Located on Spring Street in Williamstown.

Season: Year-round. **Admission:** Free. **Telephone:** (413) 458-5007.

WILLIAMS BOOKSTORE. Directions: Located on Spring Street in Williamstown. **Season:** Year-round. **Admission:** Free. **Telephone:** (413) 458-5718.

WESTERN GATEWAY HERITAGE STATE PARK. Directions: Follow Route 2 west to Route 8 south to North Adams; follow signs to park. **Season:** Year-round. **Admission:** Free. **Telephone:** (413) 663-6312. **Note:** Handicapped accessible.

NATURAL BRIDGE STATE PARK. Directions: Located on Route 8 north, ½ mile north of North Adams. **Season:** Mid-May through mid-October. **Admission:** Parking fee. **Telephone:** (413) 663-6312.

BASCOM LODGE. Directions: From Route 2 in North Adams, look for Mount Greylock State Reservation sign just west of town center. Turn left on Notch Road and continue 9 miles to the summit. **Season:** Mid-May through October. **Admission:** Free. **Telephone:** (413) 743-1591. **Note:** Mailing address is AMC Bascom Lodge, P.O. Box 686, Lanesboro, MA 01237.

For further information or restaurant and lodging suggestions, contact the Northern Berkshire Chamber of Commerce, 69 Main Street, North Adams, MA 01247. Telephone: (413) 663-3735.

NEW HAMPSHIRE

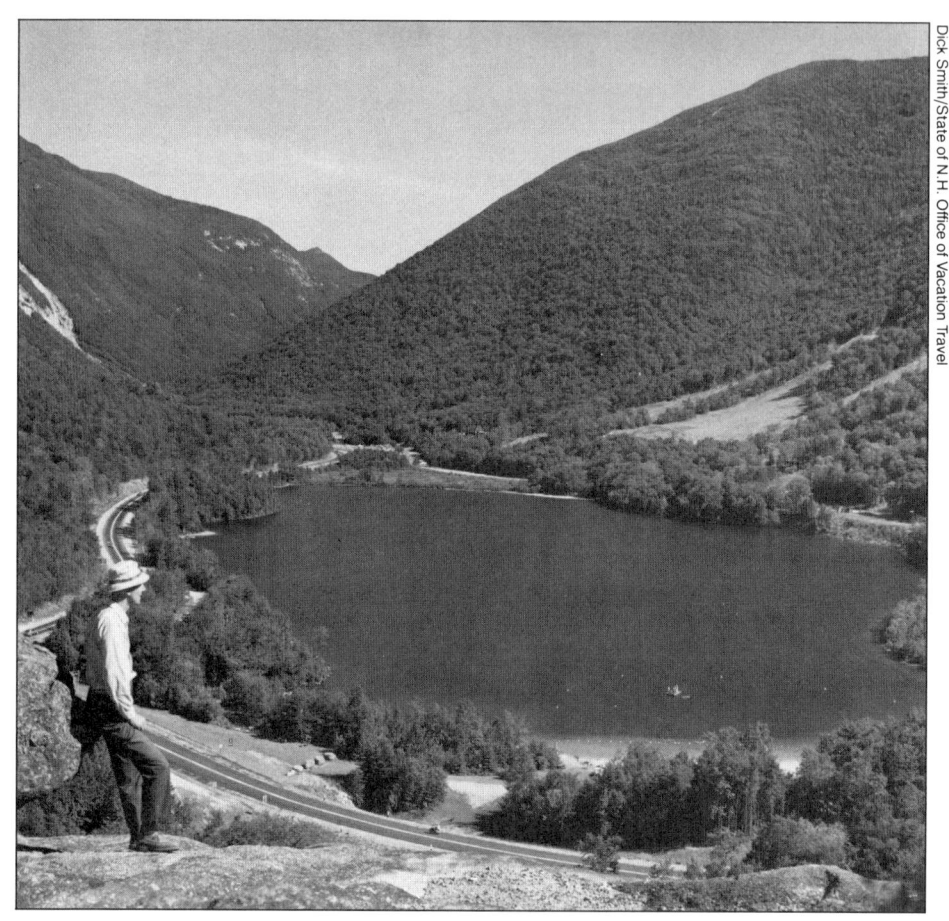

New Hampshire's expansive White Mountain National Forest abounds with pristine charm and opportunities for outdoor activities. Here a hiker pauses above Echo Lake on the northern end of the Franconia Notch Parkway.

Canterbury

You do not arrive in Canterbury by chance. Tucked away in the country, it is not really on the way to anywhere else. You have to *want* to go there. You have to have a reason, and reason there is.

You can spend the day at **Canterbury Shaker Village** learning about an unusual aspect of American history, culture, and religion in a magnificent rural setting. Add to this the elements of good conversation and good eating, and you begin to get a feel for what makes a visit to Canterbury Shaker Village a thoroughly satisfying experience. Unlike most tourist destinations, the village manages to make visitors feel like welcome guests rather than paying customers, while at the same time efficiently catering to their needs. Be sure to allow plenty of time, at least half a day, to savor the experience. Wear comfortable walking shoes and come when the weather is fair, as you will want to spend time outside as well as in.

You may have visited other "living history" villages, but none where the term applies quite so literally. Here you will be greeted by Eldress Bertha or Eldress Gertrude, two of the eight surviving Shakers (three live here and five others at the Sabbathday Lake Shaker community in Maine). Your visit begins with an informal chat with Eldress Bertha, whose parents died when she was a child and who has lived at Canterbury since 1906. The Shakers neither married nor had children, so the way the community grew was through converts and by taking in orphans who, at the age of twenty-one, could decide whether they wished to become Shakers or not. After talking a bit about her childhood, Eldress Bertha offers her blessing and sends you off for a walk through the village.

You then begin a one-and-a-half-hour guided tour that includes stops at five buildings. As you walk across one of the lush green fields, your guide will explain that the Shaker religion was founded by Mother Ann Lee, who came to this country from England in 1774. The Shakers practiced a communal lifestyle and devoted themselves to God. Sixth of the nineteen Shaker communities in the United States, Canterbury was founded in 1792. At its height, just prior to the Civil War, the community was home to between 350 and 400 members, who lived and worked in the one hundred buildings and four thousand acres that made up the community. Today the village is composed of six hundred acres and twenty-two buildings.

Your guide will discuss the way in which the Shakers' religious beliefs affected their culture. He or she will provide a liberal dose of Shaker history, commenting on inventions, crafts, furniture, and architecture. Historians recognize the Shakers for their ingenuity, and the tour provides an opportunity to see some of their inventions, including the flat broom, a seed planter worn by the farmer like a yoke, an institutional washing machine, and those famous Shaker boxes and baskets. Many original pieces are displayed in the buildings.

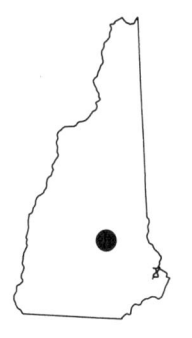

Historians recognize the Shakers for their ingenuity, and the tour provides an opportunity to see some of their inventions, including the flat broom and those famous Shaker boxes.

NEW HAMPSHIRE / 85

You'll learn all sorts of things during your walk. You'll find that the meetinghouse is completely insulated with moss and birch bark and that the Shakers wrote more than ten thousand songs and hymns. You'll also discover that the Shakers were the first to raise and package seeds commercially. Each building has a letter and each room a number, so that, for example, a child could be quickly dispatched to find the pin cushion on the second shelf of the cupboard in A6.

The tour includes a stop at the communal laundry (Eldress Bertha says she did a lot of singing while she put in her time washing and pressing clothes), with its inventive drying racks. You'll learn that the Canterbury Shakers manufactured sarsaparilla, witch hazel, and applesauce, along with hosiery, sweaters, and fancy goods. In the school building, the tour's final stop, your guide will explain that you didn't have to be a Shaker to attend what was recognized as the best school in the area. Take a look at the handwriting on the board, a perfect script courtesy of Eldress Bertha, who studied the Palmer method right in this schoolhouse.

Try to leave time in your visit to sample some Shaker culinary treats. The Summer Kitchen is the place for coffee, cookies, and a quick sandwich, which you can eat right at the kitchen table or in the pretty garden out back. The Creamery serves lunch daily in a sunny dining room with an old-fashioned ceiling fan. Enjoy some Shaker soup and a squash biscuit, or try more substantial fare, such as Shaker vegetable pie with a rice crust. For dessert, jam cake with rose water icing and cider cake with maple icing both deserve special consideration. Meals are served at long Shaker trestle tables, complete with blue place mats, pitchers of ice water, and vases of fresh flowers.

For a really special treat, join the Candlelight Dinner and Tour offered each Friday evening and some Saturday evenings throughout the season.

For a really special treat, join the Candlelight Dinner and Tour offered each Friday evening and some Saturday evenings throughout the season. The menu changes frequently, but a typical dinner might include cream of mushroom soup, a squash biscuit, a choice of baked scallops with lemon butter or roast lamb with minted sauce, a baked potato, alabaster turnip with potato, broiled herb tomatoes, honey cake with almonds, and chilled spiced cider.

Be sure to allow time to visit the attractive gift shop, where you might see a craftsperson at work making herbal wreaths or packaging sweet marjoram, lavender, dill weed, or rosemary from the village garden. The stock includes handsome reproduction Shaker baskets and oval boxes with walls made

Demonstrations of Shaker crafts add to the appeal of a visit to Canterbury Shaker Village.

of cherry and tops and bottoms of clear pine. Also available are dolls in Shaker costume, spirit drawings, stenciling supplies, crockery, tinware, fancywork, reproduction straw bonnets, and jars of honey and rose water. Shaker furniture, including trestle tables, footstools, and several types of chairs, are sold in finished or kit form.

In the adjoining workshops, you might catch a tinsmith fashioning a coffeepot, a chair maker taping a Shaker chair, or a basket maker weaving ash splints into a traditional Shaker kittenhead basket. The village also offers an annual crafts seminar each June, which combines an opportunity to feast on Shaker cookery with lectures by guest artisans, workshop tours, and hands-on experience in a given craft such as basketry or broom making. Call ahead for dates and fees.

ACCESS

CANTERBURY SHAKER VILLAGE. Directions: Traveling north on I-93, take exit 15E. Follow I-393 east for 5 miles. Turn left on Route 106 and continue north for 7 miles. Turn left on Shaker Road and continue 2½ miles to village. Traveling south on I-93, take exit 18 and follow signs to Shaker Village. **Season:** Mid-May through mid-October. **Admission:** Charged. **Telephone:** (603) 783-9511. **Note:** Reservations are required for the Candlelight Dinner and Tour.

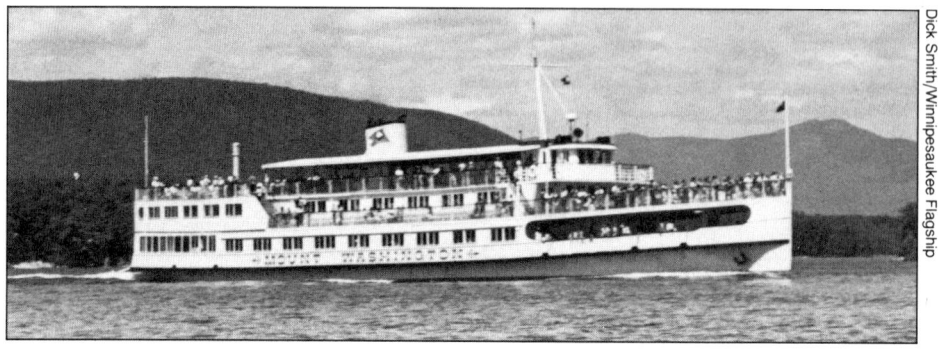

More than 1,200 passengers can sail the Mount Washington *for a tour of New Hampshire's largest lake, Lake Winnipesaukee.*

Meredith

Although it is often translated as "beautiful water in a high place," there is no firm consensus as to the origin of Lake Winnipesaukee's name. One legend holds that an Indian warrior named Kona fell in love with Ellacaya, daughter of an enemy chief, Ahanton. So impressed was the chief by Kona's bravery in asking for his daughter's hand that he permitted the marriage. Feeling optimistic as he watched Kona and Ellacaya paddle off together across the water, Ahanton is said to have proclaimed, "That all may know of the peace between us, may these waters be called winnipesaukee, the smile of the Great Spirit." All in all, there are more than one hundred legends relating to the origin of the lake's name. Whichever one you choose to believe, no doubt you'll find Lake Winnipesaukee as hypnotic and enticing as the Indians did.

Cheerful, relaxed Meredith makes an ideal base for your day or weekend by the lake. There's plenty to do within a short drive of town, or you can park your car and treat yourself to a leisurely lake cruise or a scenic railroad trip.

The best way to become acquainted with New Hampshire's largest lake is to take one of **Winnipesaukee Flagship**'s cruises. The *Mount Washington*, a 230-foot excursion ship, can accommodate more than twelve hundred passengers. Board the "Mount" at Center Harbor or Weirs Beach (it also stops at Wolfeboro and Alton Bay), both just a few miles from Meredith, for a three-and-a-quarter-hour cruise. During the fifty-mile excursion, there's ample opportunity to get a close look at some of the 274 islands — from great to very, very small — that stud Winnipesaukee's waters.

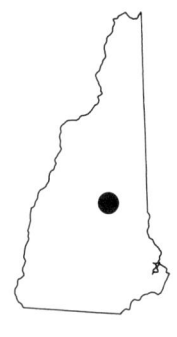

Eating is very much a part of the onboard activity. The cafeteria provides breakfast, lunch, and snacks, and there's also a comfortable restaurant with cocktail service. In addition to day cruises, the "Mount" offers romantic evening dining and dancing, with two different bands providing music on separate dance floors. Special evening "theme cruises" are held throughout the season, featuring dinner and entertainment in keeping with the evening's theme. Write ahead for a schedule so you can select from Hawaiian Luau, Dixieland Jamboree, Irish Fling, Oktoberfest, and a dozen others.

If you prefer a shorter cruise, take a one-and-three-quarter-hour ride aboard the *Sophie C* or *Doris E*, each of which has a 150-passenger capacity. The *Sophie C* is a United States mail boat. It's fun to cruise the channels and coves, delivering letters and packages to the people who live on the islands. The captain on each boat provides a lively commentary filled with stories about the history of the lake.

Another way to experience the pleasures of the lake is to take a ninety-minute cruise aboard the **Queen of Winnipesaukee,** a forty-six-foot sloop with a mast that towers fifty-eight feet above the water. It's peaceful to glide between the islands, heeling gently as the wind fills the sails, undisturbed by the constant drone of an engine. The sloop has room for fifty passengers and offers early evening and moonlight sails.

Do some Lakes Region sightseeing while giving yourself a break from the rigors of driving by taking a scenic trip aboard the **Winnipesaukee Railroad,** which runs on early-period diesel equipment. The round trip between Meredith and Lakeport takes almost two hours. For a shorter ride, get on at Weirs Beach. Take the northbound leg to Meredith and return to Weirs on the southbound leg, skimming along the banks of Meredith Bay. Total riding time is under one hour. During foliage season you can travel by train from Meredith or Weirs Beach to Plymouth, passing through the woods and skirting the shores of Lake Waukewan and Winona Lake. You'll climb the steep ascent to Ashland Summit, and scuttle across the Ashland trestle, continuing on through Pemigewasset River country en route to Plymouth, where the engine turns the train around for the return run.

If the weather takes a turn for the worse, head for **Mill Falls Marketplace,** smack-dab in the center of Meredith. Nearly twenty shops, restaurants, and boutiques occupy three stories in this renovated mill building and the several new adjacent structures built to complement it. Fine linen was originally pro-

"That all may know of the peace between us, may these waters be called winnipesaukee, the smile of the Great Spirit."

duced in the mill, built in the late 1880s following the destruction by fire of the original knit-goods mill on the same site. Manufacturing of one sort or another continued here for over two centuries. The ambiance within is strictly country casual. Outside, the pleasant landscaping includes broad brick walkways, lots of park benches, and chunky wooden barrels overflowing with flowers.

The shops specialize in everything from candy to craft supplies, from fine fashions to jewelry to antiques. There's a full-fledged, sit-down-and-stay-awhile restaurant on the first floor, but if you're in the mood for a light snack or meal, try **Upcountry Provisions & Café** on the second floor. A combination kitchen store (gourmet gadgets to fine glassware), bakery, and informal restaurant, it's a good place to satisfy your appetite any time of day. For breakfast, consider homemade muffins, Danish, or croissants. Lunch and dinner fare includes simple sandwiches and fancier offerings such as lobster salad or a gyroburger (ground lamb on Syrian bread with chopped onion, tomato, and yogurt dressing). You also can order half a sandwich with a cup of delicious homemade soup. And if you'd like to have a picnic by the lake, this is the place to assemble it.

During the summer you'll find plenty of free entertainment at the marketplace. Groups specializing in Dixieland, barbershop, folk, and country perform there. One ensemble plays favorites from Broadway to Basin Street, songs identified with Gershwin, Irving Berlin, Fats Waller, and Louis Armstrong. Entertainment is usually scheduled in the early evening on Wednesdays and Fridays, Sunday afternoons, and some Monday evenings. Pick up a schedule when you arrive.

Come Wednesday, Thursday, or Friday and treat yourself to some great classical music courtesy of the **New Hampshire Music Festival Orchestra,** which performs in Plymouth and Gilford, both less than half an hour's drive from Meredith. Since its origin in 1953 the orchestra has earned a fine reputation, and its program now includes a series of chamber music concerts in addition to its orchestral performances. For a complete schedule and ticket information, write to the festival at the business office, P.O. Box 147, Center Harbor, NH 03226.

Homage is paid to another very different sort of Lakes Region tradition at **Annalee's Gift Shop and Museum.** Annalee Thorndike has been making dolls for more than fifty years. If you or your offspring ever had an Annalee doll as a child, you'll

If you'd like to have a picnic by the lake, this is the place to assemble it.

enjoy a visit to this small museum, where the history and craftsmanship of these appealing toys is documented. A brief video introduces Annalee and her family and explains how the doll business was launched following the failure of the family egg hatchery business in the 1940s. Because her dolls can be adapted to almost any position, Annalee and her husband called them mobility dolls. Soon after Annalee began making the dolls, she started getting orders from department stores that wanted to commission dolls for window displays.

You'll see the artist's proof of Foxy Lady (1981), the face hand-painted by Annalee. Dressed fit to kill in a fur boa, pearls, and strapless gown, she fits right in with her escort, who sports a top hat, a gold cane and watch fob, and a pearl-buttoned lace shirt. There's a collection of dolls made in 1958 for Rogers Department Store in Manchester, New Hampshire, which includes a pair of scrapping little boys and a well-dressed mama pushing her baby in a stroller. A fanciful lake scene shows Annalee dolls having the time of their lives — driving motorboats, water-skiing, swimming, sunning, and just plain earning that "mobility doll" label. In another diorama, several dolls go rock climbing, while others preen for the camera. Each doll has its own distinct personality. Some of the dolls are on loan from the State of New Hampshire, and others are on exhibit courtesy of the New Hampshire State Liquor Commission.

The museum includes the Antique and Collectible Shop, where you can purchase valuable Annalee dolls (some of which were manufactured for only one year). There is also a gift shop where more recent models are sold at much more modest prices.

Whether you are a serious collector or a tourist in search of a meaningful remembrance of your vacation in New Hampshire, you'll be warmly received at **The Old Print Barn,** where Charles and Sophia Lane sell original prints spanning three hundred years, with particular emphasis on the nineteenth century and "the very contemporary." According to the Lanes, this renovated nineteenth-century barn features "rare and common, old and modern, artistic and illustrative prints of lithographs, etchings, and engravings, and all styles that the artists have created" from 1600 to the present day.

Hand-hewn pine beams serve as supports for the hundreds of pictures exhibited on the main floor and in the two lofts. Open and airy, with lots of track lighting, braided rugs on the floor, and comfortable chairs to rest in while contemplating the wealth of

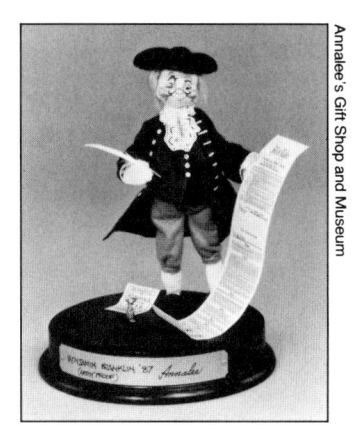

Annalee dolls have been a New England tradition since the 1940s.

prints around you, the gallery is both functional and welcoming.

In addition to a fine selection of New Hampshire subjects and works by artists from many parts of the United States, the Print Barn has prints from all over the world. And every single print is an original; no reproductions at all. The Lanes have studied fine prints for the past thirty years and for the last ten have shared their knowledge through a quarterly publication, *Journal of the Print World*. In 1986 their paper was represented at more art expositions and rare print shows than any other publication in the field. Congenial and absolutely unpretentious, they know their business inside out and are eager to share their expertise with novice as well as experienced collector. A visit to The Old Print Barn may well turn out to be a memorable highlight of your visit to Meredith.

Before leaving Meredith, enjoy lunch or dinner at **Hart's Turkey Farm Restaurant,** a long-time Lakes Region favorite. As the name suggests, turkey is the specialty. Turkey dinners come in small, regular, and jumbo portions. Then there's turkey salad, cold turkey plate, turkey nuggets, turkey chow mein, turkey croquettes, turkey livers, turkey divan, turkey Parmesan, and turkey cordon bleu, not to mention our favorite, steaming turkey pie with a puff pastry topping. But while the restaurant's name reveals its specialty, it doesn't indicate the vast number of other choices on the menu. Beef, lamb, veal, and ham dishes are available, and there's a good selection of seafood, from Alaskan king crab legs to broiled sea scallops, from butterfly shrimp to broiled haddock. Many of these dishes come in mini as well as regular-size portions. There are sandwiches and salads, too, and you can order an omelette, pancakes, or French toast any time of day.

The expansive dessert list includes Grandma Hart's cheesecake with strawberries, mocha mousse, parfaits (alcoholic and nonalcoholic), and sundaes. When it comes to the pies, it's hard to know where to begin. There's key lime, grasshopper, sawdust (pecan and coconut), chocolate chip, and about eight fruit varieties — all made right on the premises by the resident pastry chef. Suffice to say, it's wise to come to Hart's good and hungry.

ACCESS

MEREDITH. Follow I-93 to exit 23. Travel east on Route 104 to Route 3. Turn left on Route 3 and continue into Meredith.

> *A visit to The Old Print Barn may well turn out to be a memorable highlight of your visit to Meredith.*

WINNIPESAUKEE FLAGSHIP. Directions: The *Mount Washington* departs from Weirs Beach, Center Harbor, Alton Bay, and Wolfeboro. The *Sophie C* departs from Weirs Beach only, and the *Doris E* departs from Weirs Beach and Meredith. **Season:** Late May through mid-October for the "Mount"; mid-June through early September for the two smaller boats. **Admission:** Charged. **Telephone:** (603) 366-5531. **Note:** For schedule, write to Winnipesaukee Flagship, Box 367, Weirs Beach, NH 03246.

QUEEN OF WINNIPESAUKEE. **Directions:** From Meredith, follow Route 3 south to Weirs Beach. The boat is docked behind the Weirs Beach Railroad Station. **Season:** Memorial Day through Columbus Day. **Admission:** Charged. **Telephone:** (603) 524-1911.

WINNIPESAUKEE RAILROAD. Directions: Traveling south on Route 3, turn left at Ladd Hill Road opposite Hart's Turkey Farm. Railroad is on right. Or follow Route 3 south to Weirs Beach and board at the Weirs Beach station. **Season:** Late May through foliage season; limited schedule from May to late June and after Labor Day. **Admission:** Charged. **Telephone:** (603) 528-2330.

MILL FALLS MARKETPLACE. Directions: Located at the junction of routes 3 and 25 in Meredith. **Season:** Year-round. **Admission:** Free. **Telephone:** (603) 279-7006.

NEW HAMPSHIRE MUSIC FESTIVAL ORCHESTRA. Directions: Performances are held at Gilford Middle-High School in Gilford and at Silver Hall, Plymouth State College in Plymouth. **Season:** Early July through mid-August. **Admission:** Charged. **Telephone:** (603) 253-4331.

ANNALEE'S GIFT SHOP AND MUSEUM. Directions: Take I-93 to exit 23. Follow Route 104 east. Turn right on Hemlock Drive and continue to museum. **Season:** Year-round; closed the week after Christmas. **Admission:** Free for seniors. **Telephone:** (603) 279-6543.

THE OLD PRINT BARN. Directions: Follow I-93 to exit 23. Follow Route 104 east to double blinker. Turn left on Winona Road. Continue 1¾ miles to large white farm on your right. There is no sign for the Print Barn, which is attached to the farmhouse, but look for the name "Lane" on the mailbox. Large field for parking. **Season:** Memorial Day through Columbus Day; call first after Labor Day; by appointment year-round. **Admission:** Free. **Telephone:** (603) 279-6479.

HART'S TURKEY FARM RESTAURANT. Directions: Located at the intersection of Routes 3 and 104 in Meredith. **Season:** Year-round. **Admission:** Free. **Telephone:** (603) 279-6212.

For further information or restaurant and lodging suggestions, contact the Meredith Chamber of Commerce, P.O. Box 732, Dept. B, Meredith, NH 03253-0732. Telephone: (603) 279-6121.

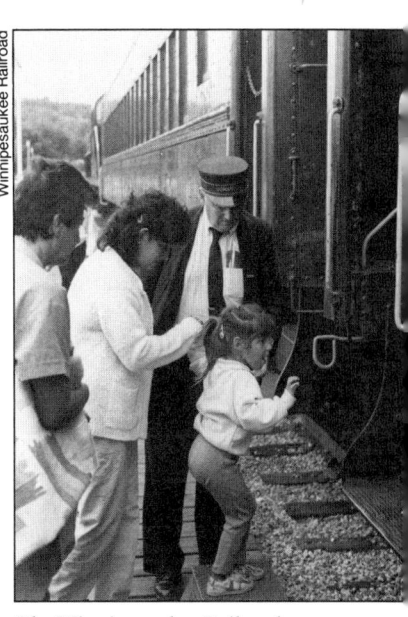

The Winnipesaukee Railroad skirts the shore of the lake on its trip from Meredith to Lakeport and back.

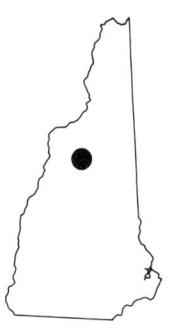

Franconia Notch

A dramatic mountain pass tucked between the Kinsman Range to the west and the Franconia Range to the east, Franconia Notch cuts through the very heart of the White Mountain National Forest. Encompassing some of the most spectacular scenery in New England, **Franconia Notch State Park** is also one of the most accessible parks in the region. The park spans the notch, under the watchful gaze of the Old Man of the Mountain, who poses serenely twelve hundred feet above Profile Lake. Yet while "Old Stone Face" still keeps guard, other aspects of the park have changed drastically in recent years. The extension of Interstate 93 through the notch has been accompanied by $20 million worth of new visitor facilities and some new rules concerning park use. The handsome new visitor center is handicapped accessible, and paved paths make it possible for wheelchair-bound persons to visit viewing areas near some of the important geologic features. The aerial tram, long a fixture here, enables almost everyone to enjoy the views from the summit of Cannon Mountain.

Get your bearings by stopping first at the **Flume Visitor Center,** where you'll pick up a brochure detailing attractions within the park and explaining how to get to them. The speed limit along the Franconia Notch Parkway is 45 mph, which is really no problem since you'll need plenty of time to take in the spectacular mountain scenery. Left turns are not permitted, which means that you have to use a series of pedestrian underpasses (park your car in the designated parking lot on the northbound side of the highway, for example, then walk underneath the road to the point of interest on the southbound side) or continue to the next interchange and reverse direction.

The visitor center, an attractive wooden contemporary building, has an information desk staffed by extremely knowledgeable, helpful park rangers. If you are unsure of your stamina and need some advice on whether to explore **The Flume,** these are the folks to consult. There are three options for viewing The Flume, but it's important to realize that all of them involve 156 steps and uphill walking. You can take a bus from the visitor center to Boulder Store, walk one-quarter mile each way to and from The Flume, and return from the store to the center by bus, with a total round-trip riding/walking time of about forty minutes. Or you can ride to the store,

The speed limit along the Franconia Notch Parkway is 45 mph, which is really no problem since you'll need plenty of time to take in the spectacular mountain scenery.

The Flume was accidentally discovered in 1808 by 93-year-old "Aunt" Jess Guernsey, who was out on a solo fishing jaunt.

walk to The Flume, and walk all the way out to the visitor center. Allow about an hour for the one-and-a-half-mile trip. The third option is to follow the graded gravel trail all the way in and all the way out. Most people take about an hour and a half to complete the hike. Whichever approach you choose, your visit to The Flume is self-guided, so you can set your own pace, and there are plenty of benches for you to rest on along the way.

The Flume itself, a natural gorge extending eight hundred feet at the base of Mount Liberty, is bordered by towering granite walls that reach skyward seventy to ninety feet. You'll walk along a boardwalk that provides a close look at the mosses, ferns, and wildflowers that thrive in this moist environment. The Flume was accidentally discovered in 1808 by ninety-three-year-old "Aunt" Jess Guernsey, who was out on a solo fishing jaunt. Her family was reluctant to believe her excited reports, but eventually they were persuaded to come and see for themselves. If you choose the second or third option mentioned above, you'll also see **The Pool,** a deep basin formed in the Pemigewasset River during the Ice Age by a silt-laden stream flowing from the glacier. A cascade rushes into The Pool, splashing over fragments of granite dislodged from the high cliffs above.

Even if you don't feel up to negotiating The Flume, there's plenty to do at the visitor center. Start by taking a look at the gracious Concord coach, a stagecoach with interior and exterior seating and leather window shades. It carried both mail and passengers through the notch for nearly half a century

NEW HAMPSHIRE / 95

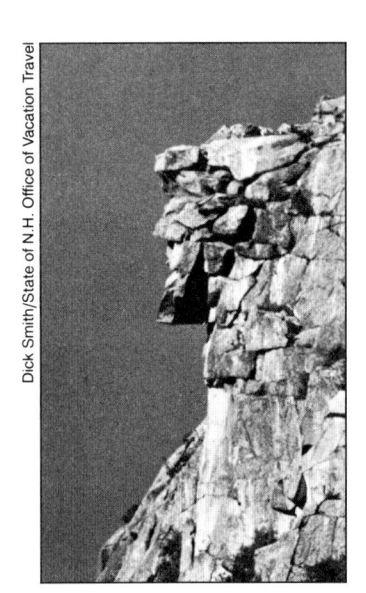

"In the mountains of New Hampshire, God Almighty has hung out a sign to show that there he makes men."

during the 1800s. Then head for the auditorium to watch the twenty-minute film introducing the park. You'll learn about the sociological and geological factors involved in the development of Franconia Notch, and you'll see some dramatic aerial photographs of the area. If others in your traveling party have opted for The Flume, leaving you to your own devices, stop in at the lively gift shop, where you can purchase a copy of *Look to the Mountain*, Le Grand Cannon, Jr.'s classic epic about an eighteenth-century couple, pioneers in the New Hampshire wilderness. Pick up a sandwich or ice cream and head for the deck leading off the cafeteria. Here you can enjoy your snack and book at a picnic table in the sun or in the shade, peacefully lulled by the sound of The Flume's water flowing past.

On leaving the visitor center, continue north to **The Basin,** where a waterfall cascades into a granite pothole twenty feet across. The rocks that make up The Basin, believed to have its origins in the Ice Age twenty-five thousand years ago, have continued to erode, smoothed away by the force of the Pemigewasset River. The water is usually about twelve feet deep at the height of summer, but even then its temperature seldom reaches fifty degrees Fahrenheit. Follow the dirt path uphill where the water bubbles through the rocks as it courses down into the rocky hole below. A paved path marked with signs leads to a handicapped-accessible viewing platform overlooking The Basin.

Continuing north through the park, you'll see signs for **Lafayette Campground,** the only place in Franconia Notch where camping is permitted. There are ninety-eight wooded tent sites, each with an open fireplace, picnic table, and parking space. Wood and charcoal are available at the campground. Running water and toilets are located near the sites, and hot showers are available in Lafayette Lodge, which also houses the registration office, the camp store, and a recreation hall where evening interpretive programs focusing on local flora, fauna, and geology are held.

Back on the road, you'll see signs for **Boise Rock,** a huge boulder with its own legend. Seems a teamster from Woodstock sought shelter beneath the great rock when he and his horse were caught in a blizzard in the early 1800s. Thomas Boise killed and skinned his horse, wrapping himself in its hide. When rescuers found him the following day, the story goes, they had to cut him free from the frozen hide that saved his life. There are picnic tables near the boulder where you can pause for a rest by a cool spring.

You don't even need to get out of the car to get a good view of the **Old Man of the Mountain,** alias "Great Stone Face" or "The Profile," although there are viewing areas where you can park and get out your binoculars. A majestic natural rock formation shaped by a series of geologic occurrences stretching back some 200 million years, the Old Man is actually five separate granite ledges forming a face about forty feet from chin to forehead. A poem attributed to Daniel Webster provides food for thought as you marvel at the profile:

> *Men hang out their signs indicative of their*
> *   respective trades:*
> *shoemakers hang out a gigantic shoe;*
> *jewelers a monstrous watch;*
> *and a dentist hangs out a gold tooth;*
> *But in the mountains of New Hampshire,*
> *God Almighty has hung out a sign to*
> *show that there he makes men.*

The Old Man overlooks Profile Lake, sometimes called the "Old Man's Washbowl." Open to fly fishing only, the small, crystalline body of water has a reputation for brook trout. Fish from its banks or launch your boat in the designated area at the south end of the lake.

You'll want to allow plenty of time for the next stop, **Cannon Tram II.** Here you can take a five-minute ride in an aerial tramway, traveling to the 4,180-foot summit of Cannon Mountain in an enclosed cable car that can hold eighty passengers. Each car has a couple of benches, although most passengers choose to stand. The tramway ascends more than two thousand feet vertically over a horizontal distance of more than a mile. The walking trails at the summit offer spectacular mountain views, and it's just a short walk to the observation deck with its fine views of neighboring Mount Lafayette, Mount Lincoln, and Mount Liberty. During the summer a naturalist is stationed at the summit to answer questions about the wildlife and plant life and to offer advice on hiking routes. There is also a cafeteria where you can refuel before boarding the tramway for the descent.

When the snow flies, the twenty-six miles of trails operated by the **Cannon Mountain Ski Area** are served by a triple chair lift, two double chair lifts, two T-bars, and a beginner's lift, in addition to the

Cannon Tram II transports passengers to the 4,180-foot summit of Cannon Mountain both winter and summer.

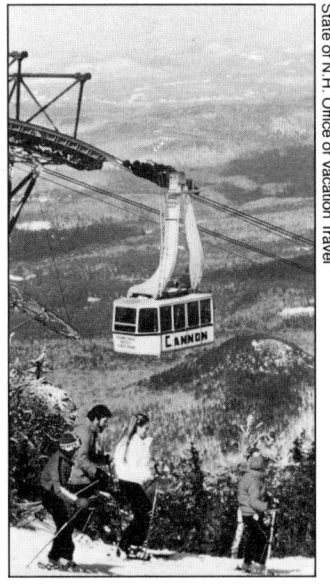

Members of the 1924 U.S. Olympic ski team (participants in the first Winter Olympics) are among those immortalized at the New England Ski Museum.

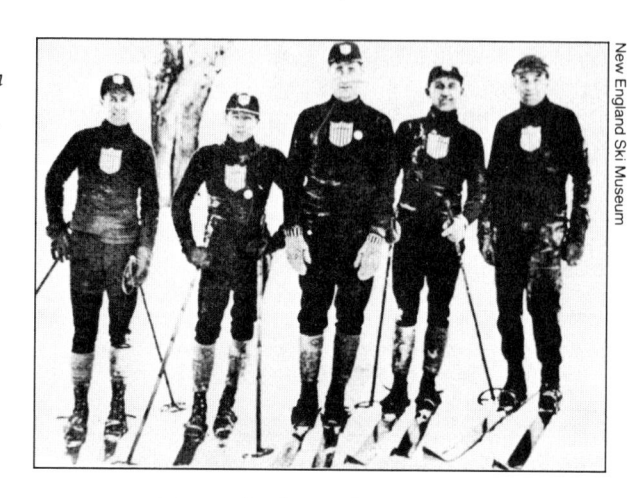

New England Ski Museum

two trams. Winter facilities also include a ski school and a ski shop.

Whether you visit in the summer, during foliage season, or in the winter, take time to stop by the **New England Ski Museum,** where you'll become familiar with the sociology and history of skiing. Beyond the artfully displayed exhibits tracing the evolution of ski equipment, the museum documents the stories of the men and women pivotal in the development of skiing as a continuously challenging recreational pursuit. The first exhibit you encounter is the dark green Cannon Mountain Tram, the first aerial passenger tramway in North America. It served skiers well from 1938 until 1980, when it was replaced by "The Lafayette," one of the trams currently serving the mountain.

A lively film documenting the history of skiing informs you that hunters in Scandinavia used skis some five thousand years ago and that the Norwegians are credited with bringing skiing to North America. The film chronicles the development of the Dartmouth Outing Club and the Lake Placid Winter Olympics, important institutions in the development of recreational skiing in the United States. The invention of the stem turn fits into the story, too, as does the evolution of the festive "ski trains" of the 1930s, which delivered carless urbanites to the mountains. You'll hear the voice of Austrian Tony Matz describing his legendary 6½-minute, 80-mph descent of the headwall at Tuckerman Ravine in 1939 when he was nineteen.

Elsewhere in the museum you'll view exhibits devoted to the story of skiing in each of the six New England states. A short self-activated slide show describes the training undertaken in the Colorado

Rockies during the winter of 1943–44 as the 10th Mountain Division, the first U.S. Army division taught to fight, climb, and ski in the mountains, prepared for service in Europe, where they were instrumental in forcing the surrender of the German forces in Italy. Another audio exhibit introduces Minnie Dole, founder of the National Ski Patrol. More than a repository for antiquated equipment, this small museum breathes life into the story of skiing and the people who made it happen.

The northernmost stop along the Franconia Notch Parkway is lovely **Echo Lake,** where you can swim or fish in the shadow of Mount Lafayette and Cannon Mountain. If you would like to set your small boat afloat, head for the Echo Lake boat launch, located beyond the Glaessel Building at Cannon Mountain.

This small museum breathes life into the story of skiing and the people who made it happen.

ACCESS

FRANCONIA NOTCH STATE PARK. Directions: Important park attractions are located along the Franconia Notch Parkway, a section of I-93 that extends eight miles, from The Flume at the southern end to Echo Lake at the northern end. **Season:** Late May through mid-October; reopens late November to mid-April for skiing.

FLUME VISITOR CENTER. Directions: Located at the southern end of the Franconia Notch Parkway. **Season:** Memorial Day through the end of October. **Admission:** Free to center; charge for The Flume; New Hampshire residents 65 years and older admitted free. **Telephone:** (603) 823-5563. **Note:** Handicapped-accessible rest rooms.

LAFAYETTE CAMPGROUND. Directions: Located on Franconia Notch Parkway. **Season:** Late May through mid-October. **Admission:** Camping fees charged. Grandparents can register with or join their families on a site at no cost beyond that charged the family. **Telephone:** (603) 823-5563 or 823-7751.

OLD MAN OF THE MOUNTAIN. Directions: View areas located along Franconia Notch Parkway, north of Lafayette Campground.

CANNON TRAM II and CANNON MOUNTAIN SKI AREA. Directions: Located on Franconia Notch Parkway. **Season:** Tram from late May through mid-October. Skiing from late November through early April. **Admission:** Charged; free to New Hampshire residents 65 years and older except on weekends. **Telephone:** (603) 825-5563. **Note:** The base lodge is handicapped accessible.

NEW ENGLAND SKI MUSEUM. Directions: Located adjacent to the Cannon Tram II. **Season:** Late May through mid-October; open for ski season late December through early April. **Admission:** Charged. **Telephone:** (603) 823-7177. **Note:** Museum is handicapped accessible.

ECHO LAKE. Directions: Exit I-93 onto Route 18 at the north end of Franconia Notch Parkway. Follow signs to parking area. **Season:** Year-round. **Admission:** Parking fee. **Telephone:** (603) 823-5563.

For further information or restaurant and lodging suggestions, contact Franconia Notch State Park, Franconia, NH 03580. Telephone: (603) 823-5563. Or contact the Office of Vacation Travel, Box 856C, Concord, NH 03301. Telephone: (603) 271-2343.

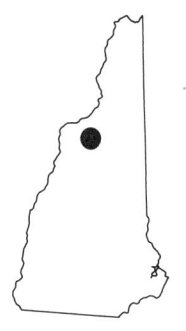

Franconia and Sugar Hill

Just a few miles beyond the border of the White Mountain National Forest, you can escape the crowds that converge on Franconia Notch and happily pass a quiet couple of days relaxing at a traditional country inn or a homey bed and breakfast. Go fishing in the local streams and ponds, go hiking on well-marked trails, or simply savor the lush rolling countryside and the splendid mountain views as you become familiar with Franconia and Sugar Hill, two small New England villages that seem to go out of their way to welcome visitors. If you are a cross-country skier, you may want to visit during winter to take advantage of the **Franconia–Sugar Hill Ski Touring Complex,** four touring centers connected by an extensive network of well-groomed trails. Write to the Franconia–Easton–Sugar Hill Chamber of Commerce for more information, including a description of the special room and board packages offered by the inns that are part of the complex.

In Franconia, allow at least an hour for your visit to **The Frost Place,** where poet Robert Frost wrote many of his best-loved poems. Your visit begins in the timbered barn, where you'll see a twenty-three-minute slide show, "Robert Frost of Franconia," describing the landscape whose influence is so consistently reflected in the poet's work. You'll also hear Frost read some of his own work.

After the show, step into the simple farmhouse where Frost lived and worked in the company of his wife and children. As his wife, Elinor, wrote in a family letter, "This house seems awfully cosy and homelike." The marble kneading board, where Mrs. Frost kneaded the family bread, sits in the upstairs bedroom now. Here you'll see hand-written letters from Frost, first editions of his works, photographs of the poet, and memorabilia such as a Morris chair fitted with a lapboard, just the kind of arrangement Frost favored when writing his poetry. You'll discover that the poet had a strong distaste for formal learning and school as a child. To compensate, his mother, a poetess, taught him at home, introducing him to poetry, history, and folklore, and in the process influencing his future.

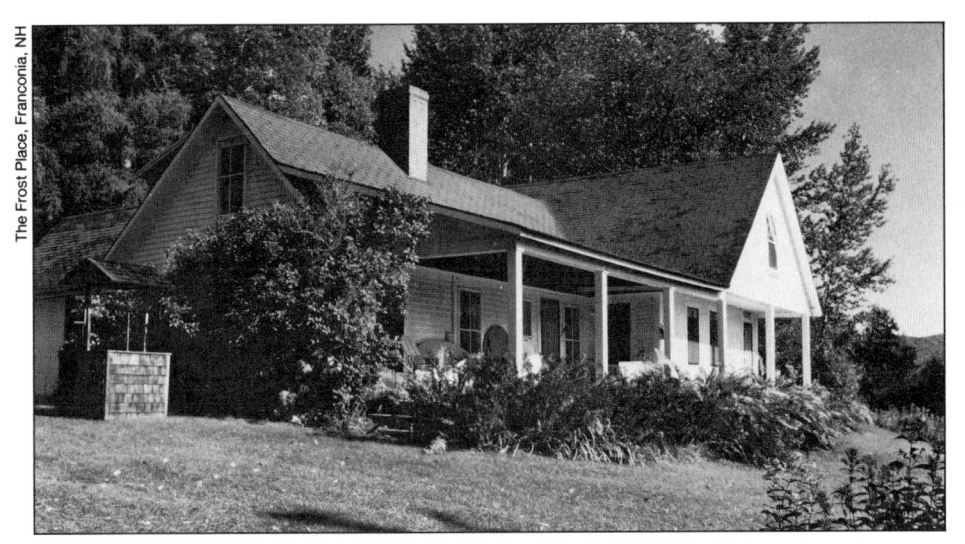

Now leave the house behind and take a leisurely walk through the woods along the poetry nature trail, which is fairly level but studded with rocks and roots. "Evening in a Sugar Orchard" and "Good-by and Keep Cold" are posted at the sites where Frost actually wrote them, and other poems are displayed where the setting seems appropriate. Read "Mending Wall" by a tumble-down stone wall overgrown with ferns and blackberries. In August the purple-fringed orchid blooms near the spot where "The Quest of the Purple-Fringed" is displayed. You'll get a glimpse of the kind of road Frost meant when he wrote "The Road Not Taken":

> *Two roads diverged in a wood, and I,*
> *I took the one less traveled by,*
> *And that has made all the difference.*

The half-mile trail begins and ends in a flower-strewn meadow with a view of the White Mountains that takes your breath away. Plants, ferns, trees, and wildflowers native to the northern New England woods are labeled, and you will be given a pamphlet describing their growing habits. Back on Main Street

Allow at least an hour in Franconia for your visit to The Frost Place, where Robert Frost wrote many of his best-loved poems.

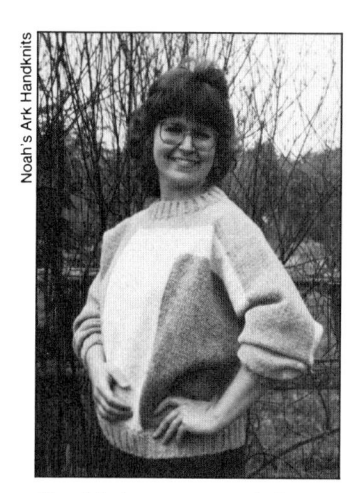

Hand-knit sweaters made from "homegrown" wool are part of the stock-in-trade at Noah's Ark in Franconia.

in Franconia, do a bit of unusual shopping. **Noah's Ark** offers a fine alternative to conventional gift shops. A cooperative founded by the Franconia Community Church of Christ to provide North Country women with a market for their handcrafts, Noah's Ark sells locally made pottery, quilts, rugs, toys, woodcrafts, and hand-knit sweaters made from wool that is "grown," dyed, and spun in New England.

Now head up the road a piece to the hamlet of Sugar Hill. Even before you enter **Polly's Pancake Parlor,** the wealth of flowers in bloom outside tells you this is a cheerful, friendly place. Located on Hildex Maple Sugar Farm in an 1830s building that was originally used as a carriage shed and later to store firewood, the dining room is decorated with antique tools, Civil War relics, old advertising posters, and sheet music covers. It seats about seventy-five hungry visitors and offers lovely views of the countryside.

Pancakes are the specialty of the house, of course, and you can eat them from breakfast through supper. Both pancakes and waffles are made from scratch with buckwheat, cornmeal, and whole wheat batter, often combined with blueberries, coconut, or walnuts. Try some of Polly's homemade country sausage or corncob-smoked bacon or ham. Your pancakes come with burnished pewter pots of maple syrup, granulated maple sugar, and thick maple spread. The menu also includes sandwiches served on homemade bread, quiches, soups, baked beans, and homemade English muffins. For dessert (after all, you're on vacation), try maple Bavarian cream or a maple hurricane sundae. The homemade pies are delicious, too.

To stretch out your vacation, take home some reminders of the good food you enjoyed on the farm. You can purchase jugs of maple syrup, naturally, but you'll also find containers of pure granulated maple sugar, perfect for sprinkling on your morning cereal or toast, and pure maple spread, wonderful on grapefruit and pancakes and a super glaze for baked ham or sweet potatoes. Or perhaps you'd like one of the six gift boxes, each containing one or more of the maple products along with some of Polly's own pancake mixes, made with organically grown grains stone-ground right here on the farm.

Come to think of it, Sugar Hill is full of good things to eat. At the **Sugar Hill Sampler,** which certainly earns its name, you'll be greeted with a free sample — hot or iced, depending on the weather —

of owner Barbara Parker's spiced tea. She packages the blend of cinnamon, orange, cloves, and other good things in small apothecary jars, should you wish to take some home. The counter is covered with larger glass jars filled with old-fashioned and imported candies such as anise drops and Swiss fruits, apricot brandy cordials and honey horehound drops. Want a sample? No problem! If that's not enough, there's even a tasting tray where you can sample jams, jellies, relishes, and mustards.

The samples, however, are only the beginning. This sprawling barn of a store also contains a museum focusing on local history, with an emphasis on the owner's family. You'll see a flouncy pink wedding dress worn by a distant ancestor, along with immense threshing baskets once used on this former farm. There's a family cradle that rocks back and forth rather than sideways and a nineteenth-century song book from the Sugar Hill Advent Church, which once was well known for its fine male chorus of forty voices. When your feet need a break, take a seat on one of the rocking chairs and leaf through some 1940s copies of *Life* magazine.

The family heirlooms are not for sale, but elsewhere in the Sampler all sorts of antiques are available: housewares, elegant paper products, baskets, candles, glassware, and much more. The stock is displayed on everything from an old wicker baby carriage to a marble-top dresser — even in a clawfoot bathtub.

Continue munching your way through Sugar Hill at **Harman's Country Store**, where the emphasis is on Cheddar, all of it aged at least two years. Other delicacies include maple syrup, twelve kinds of berry preserves, canned smoked salmon (slices and pâté), crab meat (blue crab or backfin lump), and she-crab soup. The store does a big mail-order business and these folks will gladly ship your purchases home for you. While you're here, you can browse through the shelves of used books and take a look at the handmade sweaters, hats, and mittens. In cold weather, you can warm up by the Glenwood stove before venturing back out into the elements. "People don't seem to be in much of a hurry when they come in here," observes owner Maxine Aldrich, who always offers cheese samples to her visitors.

Just across the street is the **Sugar Hill Historical Museum,** one of the more intriguing local institutions of its kind. Established in the mid-1970s with community elbow grease, the museum chronicles the evolution of life in this picturesque hilltop town.

"People don't seem to be in much of a hurry when they come in here," says the owner of Harman's Country Store.

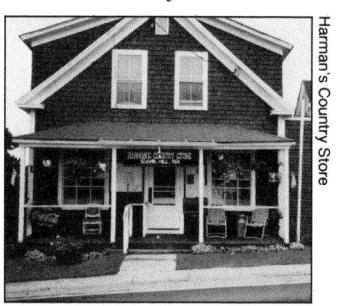

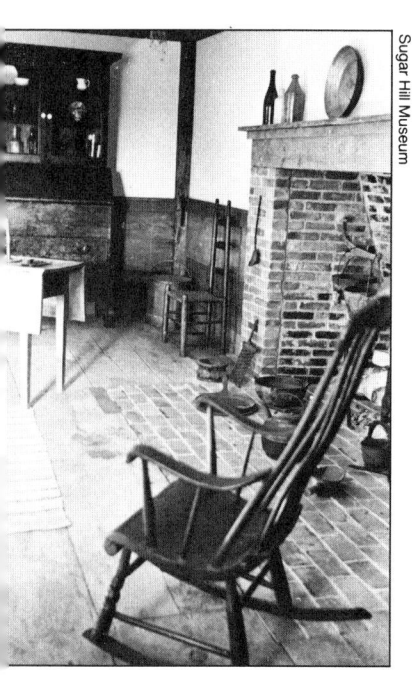

The Sugar Hill Historical Museum's Cobleigh Tavern Room re-creates a stagecoach tavern kitchen.

A hunting ground for the Abnaki Indians in its earliest days, Sugar Hill was first permanently settled by colonists who earned a livelihood as farmers. With the extension of the railroad lines, timber and iron ore became important industries. By the end of the nineteenth century, Sugar Hill saw the development of still another industry — tourism. Such periods in the community's development are interpreted in changing and permanent exhibits that include a fine collection of nineteenth-century photographs.

Take a look at the map of the Star mail routes and stage lines of Grafton County in 1885 and you'll discover that it took a two-horse conveyance one and a half hours to travel the seven and a half miles between Sugar Hill and neighboring Lisbon. Peer into a glass case displaying products made by early nineteenth-century Sugar Hill shoemaker Amos Cogswel and you'll find that a pair of calfskin shoes went for $1.50, while thick boots commanded $4. Settle down at the stereopticon with a basket of local view cards for a different look at early Sugar Hill. The Cobleigh Room, a reproduction of a stagecoach tavern kitchen, contains artifacts such as a coachman's whip and three diminutive dresses that belonged to a little girl born on a nearby farm in 1892.

Out in the barn there's an audio-visual presentation on Sugar Hill's history, as well as a display centering on the operation of the early Franconia Iron Works. A collection of horse-drawn vehicles features the handsome mountain wagon used by one of Sugar Hill's turn-of-the-century luxury hotels and the piano box sleigh that belonged to actress Bette Davis when she summered in Sugar Hill. The horse-drawn Sugar Hill hearse, built at a cost of $200 in 1890 and used until the early 1920s, is on display as well.

The museum also contains a genealogy library, featuring a complete genealogy of the early settlers of Sugar Hill, complemented by maps tracing where they settled and their subsequent marriage patterns. If you have New England roots, you may discover that some of your own forebears lived in Sugar Hill.

For a memorable summer evening, attend a performance by the **North Country Chamber Players,** an ensemble that includes musicians who play regularly at Lincoln Center and Carnegie Hall and in major concert halls throughout the world. The nineteenth-century Sugar Hill Meeting House, a simple clapboard structure complete with a graceful steeple, is a delightful setting for fine chamber music. Recent audiences have been delighted by an evening of

Viennese classics (Beethoven, Brahms, and Mozart), a Schubert concert, and a program of concertos by Vivaldi, Telemann, Albinoni, and Bach. The season lasts six weeks.

Settle down at the stereopticon with a basket of local view cards for a different look at early Sugar Hill.

ACCESS

FRANCONIA. Follow I-93 north to exit 38. Take Route 116 west, following signs into Franconia.

SUGAR HILL. From Franconia, take Route 117 two miles west to Sugar Hill.

FRANCONIA–SUGAR HILL SKI TOURING COMPLEX. Directions: Based at four different inns. Contact the Franconia–Easton–Sugar Hill Chamber of Commerce, Franconia, NH 03580, for information. **Telephone:** (603) 823-5661.

THE FROST PLACE. Directions: Take I-93 to exit 38. Follow Route 116 west for 1 mile, then follow signs to The Frost Place. **Season:** Memorial Day through Columbus Day; afternoons only. **Admission:** Charged; senior discount. **Telephone:** (603) 823-8038.

NOAH'S ARK. Directions: Located on Main Street (Route 18) in Franconia. **Season:** Mid-June through mid-October. **Admission:** Free. **Telephone:** None.

POLLY'S PANCAKE PARLOR. Directions: Located on Route 117 in Sugar Hill. **Season:** Late April through October. **Admission:** Free. **Telephone:** (603) 823-5575.

SUGAR HILL SAMPLER. Directions: Located on Route 117 in Sugar Hill. **Season:** Mid-June through October. **Admission:** Free. **Telephone:** (603) 823-5667.

HARMAN'S COUNTRY STORE. Directions: Located on Route 117 in Sugar Hill. **Season:** Year-round. **Admission:** Free. **Telephone:** (603) 823-8000.

SUGAR HILL HISTORICAL MUSEUM. Directions: Located on Route 117 in Sugar Hill. **Season:** July through late October. **Admission:** Charged; senior discount. **Telephone:** (603) 823-8142.

NORTH COUNTRY CHAMBER PLAYERS. Directions: Performances held at the Sugar Hill Meeting House, Route 117 in Sugar Hill. **Season:** Friday evenings in July and August. **Admission:** Charged; senior discount. **Telephone:** (603) 823-5392. **Note:** Call or write for a season schedule.

For further information or restaurant and lodging suggestions, contact the Franconia–Easton–Sugar Hill Chamber of Commerce, Franconia, NH 03580. Telephone: (603) 823-5661.

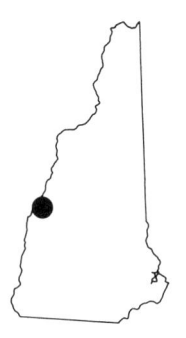

Hanover

Gracefully situated around a spacious village green that really did serve as communal grazing land two hundred years back, Hanover is the archetypal New England college town. It is most notably the home of Dartmouth College, founded in 1769 by the fiery preacher Reverend Eleazar Wheelock, "for the education of the Youth of the Indian Tribes, . . . English Youth, and any others."

Wheelock found that recruiting Indians wasn't an easy matter. Once enrolled, many failed to adjust to the type of training offered and soon dropped out. In the college's first two hundred years, only twelve Indians graduated. Yet Dartmouth eventually addressed the preacher's original mission with the establishment of a Native American studies program in the early 1970s. Currently about fifteen Native Americans graduate each year.

Today students attend class nearly year-round. A college town to the core, Hanover is the perfect setting in which to pursue your interests, be they academic or artistic. If you plan in advance, you can enroll in an intensive language course or a crafts workshop. Make your visit on the spur of the moment and you will probably find a lecture, concert, or exhibition to attend, all without leaving town.

Summer visitors should make a beeline for the information booth on the village green. Sponsored jointly by Dartmouth College and the Hanover Chamber of Commerce, the booth is usually staffed by Dartmouth alumni eager to share their enthusiasm for the college and its history, as well as for the surrounding area. This is the place to stock up on calendars of events, maps, and brochures about local attractions.

It's also the place to inquire if you wish to play golf at the Hanover Country Club, swim in the college pool, rent a canoe for a trip on the Connecticut River, play tennis, or attend a Dartmouth athletic event. If the person manning the booth doesn't have the information you need, he or she will know where to send you to get it.

The booth is also the meeting place for a free one-hour guided walking tour of the college, which begins each day from mid-June to Labor Day at 2 P.M. (Call the chamber of commerce to check the time.) You'll begin with a look at Dartmouth Row, a series of handsome white buildings with black shutters, good examples of rural Georgian architecture, even though their construction took place in the Federalist

A college town to the core, Hanover is the perfect setting in which to pursue your interests, be they academic or artistic.

period (the late eighteenth and early nineteenth centuries). Depending on the day of the week, you may visit the inside of the **Webster Cottage,** where Daniel Webster boarded during his senior year at the college. Currently headquarters of the Hanover Historical Society, the house is furnished in period pieces, some of which belonged to the famous orator.

It's just a short walk from the village green to the **Dartmouth College Hopkins Center,** which provides a lively schedule of events often featuring internationally acclaimed musicians, theater companies, and dance troupes. Students and faculty members also present their work here regularly, and an eclectic selection of films is shown in both the Spaulding Auditorium and the Lowes Theatre. Stop in at the box office to find out what events are scheduled and to purchase tickets.

The "Hop" also houses art galleries and open studios, along with the Courtyard Café, a pleasant cafeteria-style restaurant with both indoor and outdoor seating. The café serves breakfast, lunch, and dinner, and the fare is hearty and inexpensive, including muffins, bagels, chili, chowder, fried clams, pizza, salads, and sandwiches.

Another college highlight is the **Hood Museum of Art,** opened in 1985, which adjoins the Hopkins Center. To quote *Architectural Record* (February 1986), "One experiences the Hood as an unfolding sequence of pathways, nooks, and open spaces, like glimpses of a medieval landscape or interiors in a Dutch painting.... Depending on the perspective from which one views it, the Hood vaguely resembles an outpost of the late Roman Empire, a Romanesque monastery or (seen against the backdrop of a

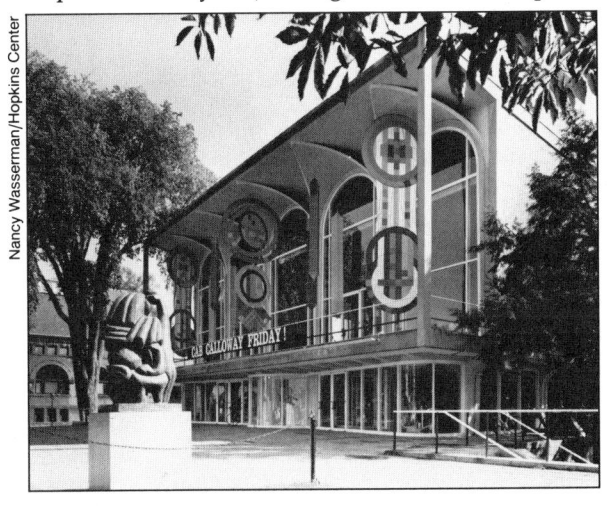

Depending on the day of the week, you may visit the inside of the Webster Cottage, where Daniel Webster boarded during his senior year at the college.

Dartmouth's Hopkins Center hosts a wealth of cultural events, including music, theater, dance, and more.

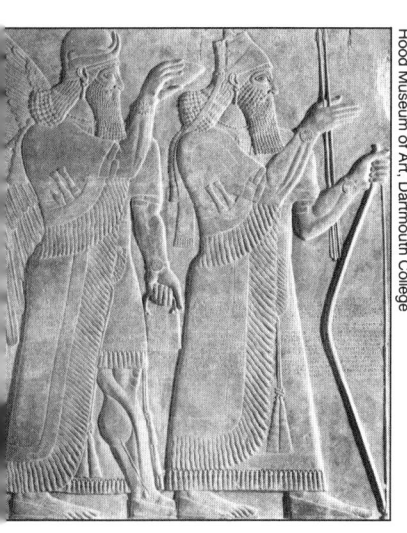

This is one of six Assyrian reliefs permanently displayed in a specially designed gallery at Dartmouth's Hood Museum of Art.

Hood Museum of Art, Dartmouth College

nearby smokestack) a nineteenth-century New England mill."

The gallery beyond the lobby — the only space in the museum planned to permanently house a specific work of art — features the museum's rarest treasure, a set of six Assyrian reliefs. They come from the palace built by King Ashurnasirpal II (883–859 B.C.) in the ancient capital city of Nimrud in what is today northern Iraq. Subjects include *The King's Attendant* (two slabs), *The King Followed by a Genie, Genie with Pail and Date-Palm Spathe, Wingless Genie with Pail and Winged Genie with Pail,* and *Genie Anointing a Sacred Tree.* Together they provide great insight into the official and ritualistic aspects of Assyrian culture.

Although the specific exhibits change, other galleries are devoted to American, Indian, European, African, and twentieth-century art. A recent show called "The Second Stage of Modernism, Art from 1945 to the Present," featured *Shards III,* an immense contemporary work by Frank Stella. The artist worked in oil, fluorescent alkyd, and epoxy on fiberglass, adding dramatic three-dimensional projections of metal and fiberglass. In sharp contrast, another gallery offered "Patterns of Life, Patterns of Art," an exquisite collection of Native American artifacts mostly from the Plains and northern woodlands tribes of the late nineteenth and early twentieth centuries.

For a look at another of the college's art treasures, stop in at the **Baker Library,** which houses Dartmouth's humanities and social sciences collections. Take the stairs just beyond the information desk down to the basement for a look at the Orozco Frescoes, a series of murals painted by Mexican artist José Clemente Orozco from 1932 to 1934, while he was artist-in-residence at the college. Orozco chose as the theme of his work "An Epic of American Civilization." In it he explores major aspects of American culture, stretching from the prehistoric migrations of primitive tribes to twentieth-century intellectual and spiritual aspirations.

To help visitors comprehend and appreciate the many ideas expressed in the murals, the library provides a free leaflet titled "An Interpretation of the Orozco Frescoes," prepared by Churchill P. Lathrop, Professor of Art Emeritus at Dartmouth. The same information is available on a tape cassette that the library will lend you along with a tape player.

When you walk away from the library, take a look at the weather vane on top of the building.

You'll see Eleazar Wheelock and a Native American student beneath a white pine, which memorializes the first Dartmouth College classroom — the ground beneath one of those towering trees so prevalent here.

As you continue to explore the campus, you may find yourself wishing you could be a student again. Well, you can. The only problem with enrolling in **ALPS** (All Language Programs) is that you'll probably be so busy you won't have time to enjoy all that Hanover has to offer. (Of course, the way to solve that dilemma is simply to extend your stay a day or two, either before or after the course.) ALPS is a ten-day intensive language program offered in the summer for beginning, intermediate, and advanced level students in French, Chinese, German, Italian, Japanese, Modern Greek, Russian, Spanish, and English as a second language.

ALPS features the Rassias method of language instruction, developed by Dartmouth professor John A. Rassias, who serves as program director. As the program brochure explains, "Participants eat, sleep, walk, run, speak solely in the language." During the ten days you'll receive a hundred hours of instruction, including small group sessions and master classes taught by Dartmouth faculty and educators trained in the Rassias method. You'll live in a college dormitory with other program participants and take your meals together at language tables.

Many different sorts of students are drawn to the ALPS program, including language teachers who want to learn elements of the Rassias method and business executives who need to acquire language skills in a limited amount of time. The program has proven particularly popular with retired people who now find that they have the time to travel abroad. Participants enjoy access to all the college recreational and cultural facilities during their stay on campus.

Hanover's Main Street is filled with attractive stores, and you're sure to find your own favorites. If you prefer gift shops to museums, do your souvenir shopping at the **Hanover League of New Hampshire Craftsmen,** where you will find handmade functional and decorative pieces produced by the cream of New Hampshire's craftspeople. A strong jury system ensures a level of quality that eliminates the tacky or distasteful. With its bare brick walls, track lighting, and front wall made of glass, the two-story shop seems more like a gallery than a store. The collection includes pieced quilts, rag rugs, rock-

You'll find only the finest juried crafts at League of New Hampshire Craftsmen shops, including one in Hanover.

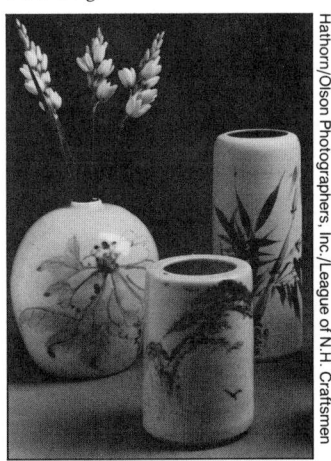

ing chairs, trestle tables, pottery, jewelry, prints, toys, woven clothing, and much more, some of it contemporary in spirit and some traditional.

The shop also offers a series of one- and two-day workshops where you can try your hand at a new technique. Recent sessions have centered on Japanese paper making, rag baskets, and melon baskets made with wild grapevines. Some workshops require previous experience. Write ahead for a calendar covering the season when you plan to visit.

Whatever your tastes, you're likely to find something delicious to order at **Molly's Balloon, Ltd.,** which combines a delicatessen and restaurant. Located right in the middle of town, Molly's is a cheerful place, decorated with lots of brass and greenery, and it draws a lively mix of students, townspeople, and visitors. Molly's menu runs the gamut from Mexican specialties such as enchiladas and fajitas to seafood entrées such as shrimp and scallop creole, as well as hamburgers and great big sandwiches. The Reuben (Bavarian kraut, corned beef, Swiss cheese, and Russian dressing grilled on rye) quickly won our approval. Desserts tend toward the rich, fattening, and intriguing. Molly's Saucy Bananas consists of bananas sautéed in Kahlua with walnuts and raisins, served hot over vanilla ice cream. If you want to put together a picnic, the adjoining deli is the perfect place to do it.

Before leaving Hanover, don't miss one more attraction, about a mile out of town. Chock-full of hands-on exhibits, the **Montshire Museum of Science** is the perfect place to take a grandchild (not that adults need any excuse). In the outdoor physics playground, you can manipulate levers to fill cylinders of different diameters with water. Before you know it, you'll be an expert on the Bernoulli effect (the pressure of moving water depends on the speed of its flow). Inside exhibits change frequently, but you'll always find an active colony of female farmer ants from South America. They live in a network of transparent tubes and blocks that look like a Le Corbusier design.

In addition to the exhibits, the museum sponsors lots of workshops and excursions. These vary from "Build a Better Boomerang" with Eric Darnell (ranked second in the world in boomerang throwing) to a day-long introduction to orienteering, and from early morning guided bird walks to an official butterfly count (held in cooperation with the Xerces Society, an organization dedicated to the conservation of rare and endangered insects). Special programs are held on Tuesday evenings throughout the fall, winter, and spring. These include lectures, films, slide shows, and demonstrations on topics ranging from the history of weather observation to stargazing, from bionics to bird psychology.

ACCESS

HANOVER. Follow I-91 to exit 13. Take Route 120 east into Hanover, arriving at village green.

WEBSTER COTTAGE. Directions: Located on North Main Street in Hanover. **Season:** Mid-June through mid-October; limited hours. **Admission:** Donation requested. **Telephone:** (603) 646-3371.

DARTMOUTH COLLEGE HOPKINS CENTER. Directions: Located adjacent to the Hanover Inn on West Wheelock Street, across from the village green. **Season:** Year-round. **Admission:** Free; tickets required for specific events. **Telephone:** (603) 646-2422.

HOOD MUSEUM OF ART. Directions: Museum is connected to the Hopkins Center. **Season:** Year-round. **Admission:** Free. **Telephone:** (603) 646-2808.

BAKER LIBRARY. Directions: The library faces Wentworth Street and the village green. **Season:** Year-round. **Admission:** Free. **Telephone:** (603) 646-2560.

ALL LANGUAGE PROGRAMS (ALPS). Information: Write to Language Outreach–ALPS, Wentworth Hall, Dartmouth College, Hanover, NH 03755. Program runs from late June to mid-July. **Telephone:** (603) 646-2922.

HANOVER LEAGUE OF NEW HAMPSHIRE CRAFTSMEN. Directions: Located at 13 Lebanon Street in Hanover, directly behind the Hopkins Center. **Season:** Year-round. **Admission:** Free. **Telephone:** (603) 643-5050.

MOLLY'S BALLOON, LTD. Directions: Located at 47 South Main Street. **Season:** Year-round. **Admission:** Free. **Telephone:** (603) 643-2570.

MONTSHIRE MUSEUM OF SCIENCE. Directions: From the village green in Hanover, follow Route 10 toward Lyme. The museum is located on your right, about 1 mile out of town. (New facility is scheduled to open in late 1988, in Norwich, Vermont, along the Connecticut River. Be alert for signs.) **Season:** Year-round; September through May closed Mondays. **Admission:** Charged. **Telephone:** (603) 643-5672.

For further information or restaurant and lodging suggestions, contact the Hanover Chamber of Commerce, P.O. Box A-105, Hanover, NH 03755. Telephone: (603) 643-3115.

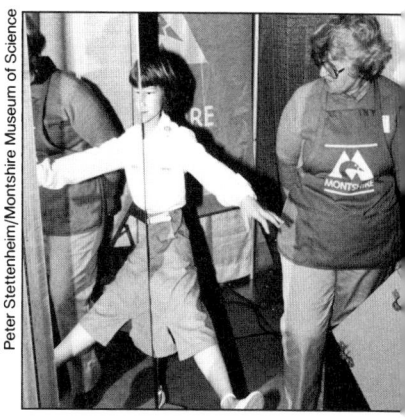

Chock-full of hands-on exhibits, the Montshire Museum of Science is the perfect place to take a grandchild (not that adults need any excuse).

VERMONT

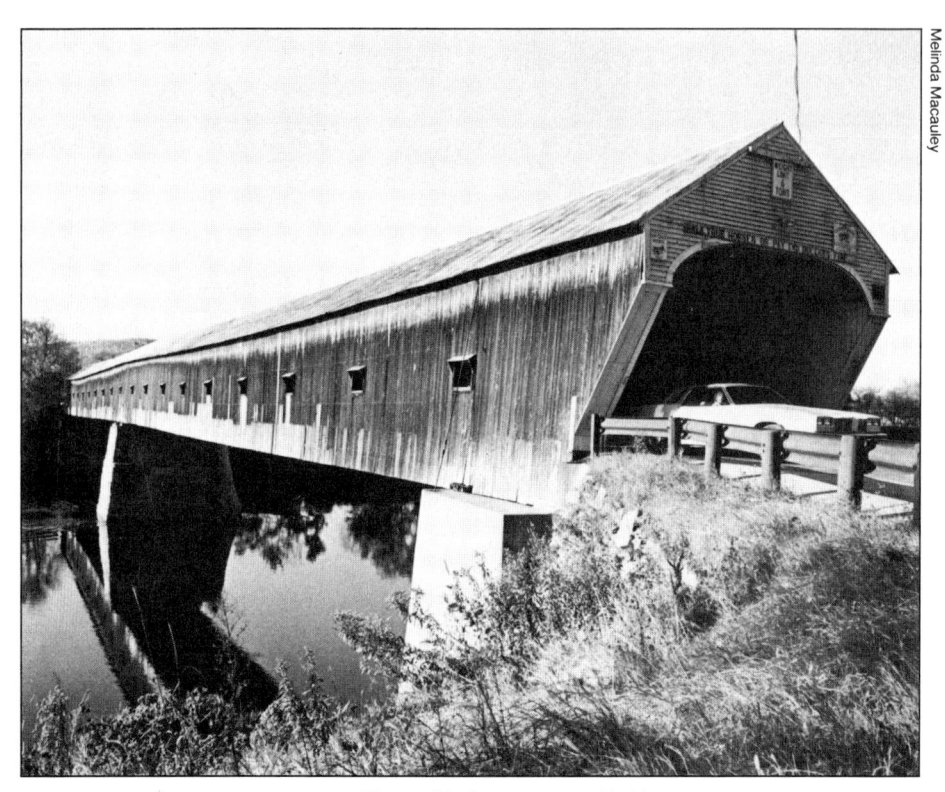

The world's longest covered bridge connects Windsor, Vermont, and Cornish, New Hampshire. Built in 1866, it was designated a National Historic Engineering Landmark in 1970.

Route 30: Brattleboro to Townshend

For an old-fashioned drive in the country, complete with simple, old-fashioned pleasures, you can't do better than spend a day exploring Route 30 between Brattleboro and Townshend. The distance is only seventeen miles — plus a few extra for any sidetrips you choose to take — yet the variety of things to do is impressive. Pick fresh produce in a sun-warmed meadow, go antiquing, try your luck at the flea markets, sample Vermont food specialties, swim or canoe in a reservoir, attend a local fair or festival. Most of all, just enjoy taking your time as you discover the West River Valley, a beautiful slice of countryside.

Begin your discovery in Brattleboro at the southern end of Route 30. A cruise aboard the mahogany-trimmed, canopy-covered *Belle of Brattleboro* is a pleasant way to become acquainted with the scenery along the Connecticut River. Your captain will tell you stories about the river and area history (the *Belle*'s dock is very near Fort Dummer, Vermont's first settlement), and point out the loons and herons that often dive and wade near the river's banks, as he navigates the forty-nine-passenger craft through the twists and turns.

A trip aboard the *Belle* is fun in the summer, when children swing on ropes from the oak trees overhanging the riverbank and the wildflowers are in bloom, but it is spectacular in the fall when the foliage is at its peak and the air is crisp and cool. There are both sunset and afternoon cruises, each lasting about one and a half hours. Simple refreshments are available, and you are welcome to bring a picnic. Arrive twenty minutes prior to sailing time and the crew will even set up an onboard table for you. Sunday morning brunch cruises and Saturday evening dinner cruises include live music.

Continuing north on Route 30, consider detouring to **Hickin's Mountain Mowings Farm and Greenhouses.** More than a hundred fruits and vegetables are cultivated here atop Black Mountain, where they are sold fresh and transformed into sweet and spicy condiments and sauces, pickles, jams, and jellies. Homemade doughnuts and bread are available, too, not to mention nearly two dozen kinds of fruit pie. Absolutely fresh-cut Christmas trees, roping, and wreaths are available in December, but you need to be a hearty soul (maybe even a hearty soul with a four-wheel-drive vehicle) to venture up to the farm after the snow flies.

Returning to Route 30, you'll soon see a sign for the **Newfane Antiques Center,** on your right. Twenty dealers set up their wares here on three floors. We saw everything from postcards (divided by subject into earthquakes, bridges, states, etc.) and old hats to Depression glass, autograph books, and a cranberry hand-blown opalescent water set consisting of six perfect tumblers and a pitcher with a fluted rim. There was quite a lot of furniture, too, from a lovely two-piece corner cupboard dating back to the early 1800s to a Victorian era walnut platform rocker upholstered in blue velvet. It's a pleasant place to

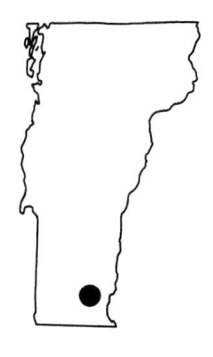

Twenty dealers display their wares at the three-story Newfane Antiques Center.

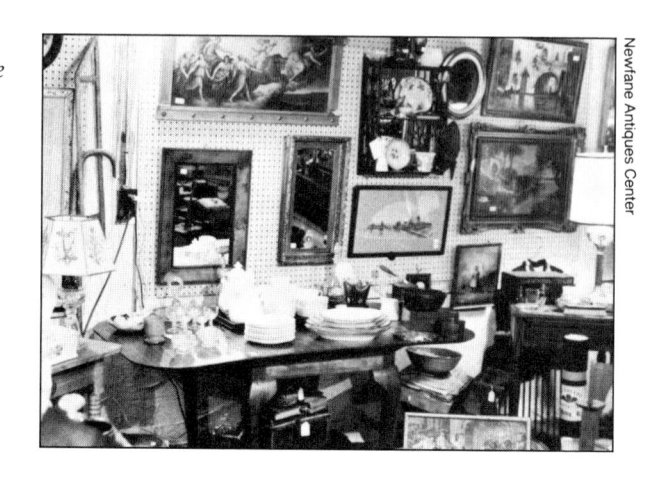

Newfane Antiques Center

This is a particularly good place to visit if you have roots in Vermont and want to do some genealogy research.

browse, especially on a winter day when you don't feel like getting in and out of the car for a few minutes here and there at the smaller shops.

Make your next stop the **Dutton Farm Stand,** where you can buy fresh Vermont produce in a sprawling wooden structure. The raspberries are ready in July, and they are something special. If you would rather harvest your own produce, venture a few miles farther north to the **Dutton Berry Farm,** where you can pick your own berries from seven in the morning until seven at night. In hot weather, an early morning or early evening visit makes sense.

Continuing now to Newfane Common, you'll arrive at a brick building with seven marble steps and a huge bell hanging in the front yard. This is the home of the **Historical Society of Windham County,** which maintains a small museum devoted to local history. This is a particularly good place to visit if you have roots in Vermont and want to do some genealogy research. Exhibits vary from year to year.

Overlooking the common itself is the **Newfane Inn.** Gnarled grapevines wrap around the woodwork above the front porch, where a neat row of green-and-white rocking chairs overlooks shoulder-high banks of pink phlox. The inn serves dinner only, and it's just the right place to dine if you want to round out your day with an elegant meal in a classic old New England inn. Children over seven are welcome, which is another way of saying "no small kids, please," ensuring a certain level of tranquility in the dining room.

The menu features elegant appetizers including pâté of venison with Cumberland sauce and home-smoked filet of trout with sauce Anglaise. Entrées include king crab flambé aux champignons and

Long Island duckling au Cointreau à l'orange or au poivre vert. Finish up with meringues glacées, coupe aux marrons, or one of the four flaming desserts. Or sip on Café Newfane Inn, a glorious mélange of coffee, Tia Maria, and whipped cream.

Just across the street you can get a feel for what's happening in town by reading the bulletin board outside the **Newfane Store,** adjacent to the common. You might find a church supper you'd like to attend, or a concert, country fair, auction, or horse-pulling contest. The big white clapboard store sells sandwiches, cheese, pickles, fruit, and just about anything you might need for a casual lunch. There are even a couple of tables out front where you can settle to consume your purchases.

A few yards away stands the 160-year-old **Newfane Country Store,** with its bare rough wood floors and heavy wooden beams. The people here make their own cream and butter fudge in eighteen irresistible flavors, such as chewy praline and vanilla walnut. There's also a great rounded glass-front candy case, as well as dozens of apothecary jars filled with delicious sweets. The store, which is absolutely packed with country crafts and New England products, also serves as headquarters for a burgeoning cottage industry. Fifty-two Vermont women sell their quilts here. You'll find hand-quilted, hand-stenciled, and hand-tied quilts, in both traditional patterns such as Log Cabin and Virginia Star and contemporary designs such as fanciful animals on a baby coverlet. Whether you are interested in a full-size quilt, a baby quilt, a wall hanging, or a pillow, you'll find a rich selection to ponder.

This is a good place to stock up on mustards, marmalades, jams, and honeys. As a matter of fact, if you look hard enough, you'll find just about anything you can imagine. A soapstone sink holds books, an old wooden freezer houses cold drinks, and a keg is filled with catnip. Just don't be surprised if a black Labrador walks in and wants to be scratched or if the blue parakeet starts singing. After all, they live here.

Continuing north of the common, pick up some succulent smoked ham, bacon, or cheese right where it's made. **Lawrence's Smokehouse** prides itself on continuing the Native American tradition of smoking only with corncobs, just as the colonists learned from the Indians. Each ham receives the traditional "cold" smoking method, which means that instead of the ten- to twelve-hour procedure used on most mass-produced hams, these are smoked at lower

Lawrence's Smokehouse prides itself on continuing the Native American tradition of smoking only with corncobs, just as the colonists learned from the Indians.

temperatures for a full week. Only mellow northern Flint corncobs (no hardwoods) are used for fuel.

Adjacent to the smokehouse is the small rustic showroom that smells deliciously of the smoked products that line its shelves and refrigerators. In addition to the bacon and ham, there's smoked Alaskan salmon and honey-cured, air-dried, and corncob-smoked boneless Idaho rainbow trout. Well over a dozen smoked cheeses, including five varieties of corncob-smoked, low-cholesterol cheese are available. Vermont Cheddar (nonsmoked) and Vermont maple syrup are available, too. Lawrence's is set up to do mail-order, so if you're going to be on the road for a spell, you can have your purchases shipped home.

Just past Lawrence's Smokehouse, you'll come to the **Newfane Flea Market,** a must if you're traveling on a Sunday. About two hundred dealers congregate in this sunny field to peddle their used, old, and absolutely antique merchandise. There's even a special section carrying automotive items — everything from parts and accessories to cars, trucks, motorcycles, and boats. Refreshments are available, and there's plenty of parking in a nearby field.

Up the road in Townshend, you can try your bargaining skills at a much smaller event. The **Townshend Flea Market** includes about twenty dealers, and the atmosphere is less hectic than in Newfane. It takes place in the **Townshend Family Park,** which also has a miniature golf course and an ice cream concession that sells "The Real Scoop," genuine, made-in-Vermont ice cream. About half the forty flavors are available at any one time. Orange coconut and Vermont apple spice certainly deserve some attention. Sundaes, milk shakes, floats, and banana splits are served up along with the ever-popular ice cream cone.

At the park you can buy some souvenirs at **Winterset Designs,** an attractive gift shop featuring lots of locally made items, including the store's own line of reasonably priced small wooden furnishings. You'll find folding tables in solid oak or cherry, cutting boards in animal shapes, and northern white cedar gardening baskets that turn silvery if left outside to weather. Other items on display include handwoven rugs from the Blue Mountains, handsome wooden lawn furniture made by Indians in Quebec, and soapstone bun warmers. Come Christmas the stock increases dramatically, making it a fruitful and cheerful place to find some out-of-the-ordinary gifts.

If you've decided to camp in the area or if you

Just past Lawrence's Smokehouse, you'll come to the Newfane Flea Market, a must if you're traveling on a Sunday.

feel like a hearty hike, stop by **Townshend State Park.** This is a pretty, quiet campground where some of the thirty-four tent sites overlook a rushing mountain stream. (Small motor homes can be accommodated on a limited basis, but there are no hookups.) Skunks and raccoons are frequent guests, so be sure to secure your food supply.

If you're in good shape and feeling particularly energetic, take the three-mile hiking trail up Bald Mountain, where you'll be rewarded with views of Bromley and Stratton mountains, and New Hampshire's Mount Monadnock, as well as the West River Valley. The round trip takes at least three hours, depending on your pace, and the resident ranger will be glad to offer suggestions for less arduous walks.

On your way to **Townshend Dam Recreation Area,** you might want to photograph **Scott's Covered Bridge,** the longest single-span covered bridge in the state. Built in 1870, it crosses the West River. You'll have to drive over the top of the dam to get to Townshend Lake and the recreation area, enjoying the dramatic view of the water far below. The swimming area features a sandy beach with easy access to the water. You can launch your own small boat here or rent a canoe, paddle boat, Sailboard, or sailboat at the **West River Canoe Center,** located right next to the beach. You can rent by the hour or by the day.

While any time in the late spring, summer, or fall is a good time to visit Townshend, you might like to know about a few special events. **Grace Cottage Hospital Fair Day** is held the first Saturday in August on the common. The fair offers tables of baked goods, crafts, and rummage. There's also an auction under a tent, a chicken barbecue, and an evening band concert. What sets this fair apart from every other country fair is the "birthday parade," when everyone born at Grace Cottage Hospital — from the time it opened in 1949 to the present — joins the much-loved country doctor who presided at their births for a march around the common.

Two other yearly events to keep in mind are the **Annual Horseshoes Tournament,** an amateur event held the second weekend in September, and the **Pumpkin Festival,** held on the common the weekend before Halloween.

Any time in the late spring, summer, or fall is a good time to visit Townshend.

ACCESS

BRATTLEBORO. Follow I-91 to exit 1, Brattleboro.

NEWFANE AND TOWNSHEND. Travel north on Route 30 from Brattleboro.

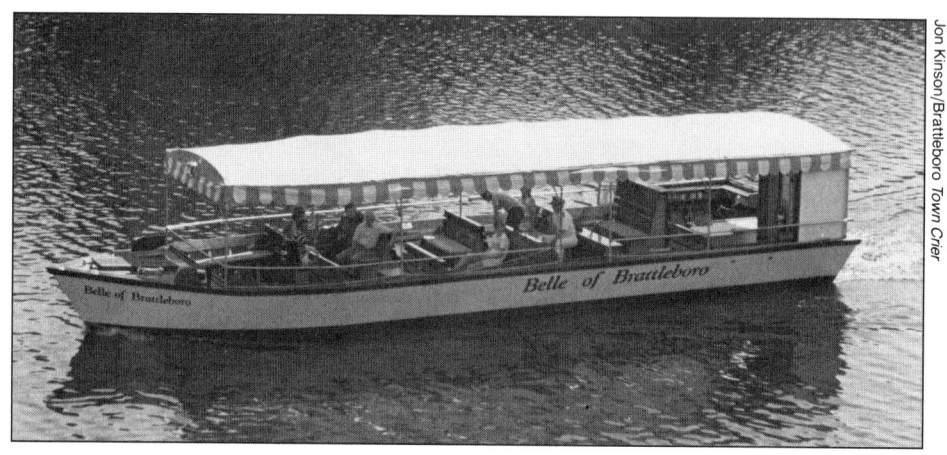

Belle of Brattleboro *cruises along the Connecticut River feature spectacular scenery during fall foliage season.*

BELLE OF BRATTLEBORO. Directions: Follow I-91 to exit 1, Brattleboro. After 1½ miles, turn right onto Route 142 south for 1 mile, then turn left on Erving Paper Company access road and follow sign to *Belle of Brattleboro*. **Season:** Memorial Day through Columbus Day; call for reservations during foliage season. **Admission:** Charged. **Telephone:** (802) 254-8080.

HICKIN'S MOUNTAIN MOWINGS FARM AND GREENHOUSES. Directions: Traveling north on Route 30 from Brattleboro, turn right on East/West Road. Bear right after crossing covered bridge. Continue until you come to Black Mountain Road on your right. Turn right and continue to farm. **Season:** Year-round. **Admission:** Free. **Telephone:** (802) 254-2146.

NEWFANE ANTIQUES CENTER. Directions: Located on Old Route 30 in Newfane Village. Continue north on Route 30 from Brattleboro toward Newfane, turning right at sign. **Season:** Year-round. **Admission:** Free. **Telephone:** (802) 365-4482.

DUTTON FARM STAND. Directions: Located on Route 30 about 1 mile south of Newfane Village. **Season:** April through December. **Admission:** Free. **Telephone:** (802) 365-4168.

DUTTON BERRY FARM. Directions: Turn right off Route 30 north at the Newfane Flea Market (below). Continue to farm entrance on your right. **Season:** Late June through July. **Admission:** Free. **Telephone:** (802) 365-4168.

HISTORICAL SOCIETY OF WINDHAM COUNTY. Directions: Located in the center of Newfane Village on Route 30. **Season:** Memorial Day through Labor Day; limited hours. **Admission:** Donation requested. **Telephone:** (802) 365-4148.

NEWFANE INN. Directions: Located on Route 30 in Newfane Village. **Season:** Year-round. **Admission:** Free. **Telephone:** (802) 365-4427.

NEWFANE STORE. Directions: Located on Route 30 in Newfane Village. **Season:** Year-round. **Admission:** Free. **Telephone:** (802) 365-7775.

NEWFANE COUNTRY STORE. Directions: Located on Route 30 in Newfane Village. **Season:** Year-round. **Admission:** Free. **Telephone:** (802) 365-7916.

LAWRENCE'S SMOKEHOUSE. Directions: Located on Route 30 in Newfane Village. **Season:** Year-round. **Admission:** Free. **Telephone:** (802) 365-7751.

NEWFANE FLEA MARKET. Directions: Located on Route 30 one mile north of Newfane Village. **Season:** May through October; Sundays. **Admission:** Free. **Telephone:** (802) 365-4000.

TOWNSHEND FLEA MARKET. Directions: Located in the Townshend Family Park. **Season:** May through October; Sundays. **Admission:** Free. **Telephone:** (802) 365-7935.

TOWNSHEND FAMILY PARK. Directions: Located on Route 30 just north of the center of Townshend. **Season:** May through October; gift shop stays open for Christmas season. **Admission:** Free. **Telephone:** (802) 365-4711.

TOWNSHEND STATE PARK. Directions: Follow Route 30 north from Newfane. Turn left at sign for park. **Season:** May through Columbus Day. **Admission:** Charged. **Telephone:** (802) 365-7500.

TOWNSHEND DAM RECREATION AREA. Directions: Located on Route 30 north of the center of Townshend. **Season:** Mid-May through mid-September. **Admission:** Free. **Telephone:** (802) 365-7500.

WEST RIVER CANOE CENTER. Directions: Located at the Townshend Dam Recreation Area. **Season:** Mid-May through mid-September. **Admission:** Rental fees charged. **Telephone:** (802) 896-6209.

For further information or restaurant and lodging suggestions, contact the Brattleboro Area Chamber of Commerce, 180 Main Street, Brattleboro, VT 05301. Telephone: (802) 254-4565.

Windsor

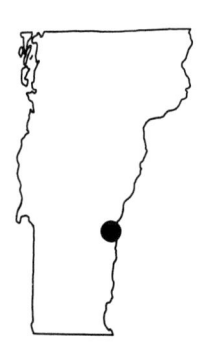

A small Vermont town that appears on the surface very much like many other small New England towns, Windsor has two claims to fame. It bills itself as the birthplace of Vermont and also as the place where the machine tool industry, born in France, was reborn. Windsor exhibits an unusual reverence for the past. Its museums and restored buildings celebrate fine craftsmanship, industriousness, and a firm adherence to democratic principles. Over the past decade the town has worked to ensure its identity in the future by supporting institutions that affirm its past. It's reassuring to visit a town where traditional values are still much respected.

The township of Windsor was formed in 1761. Many of the early settlers felt they should unite with New York, while others favored a union with New Hampshire. A third group argued for the formation of a new state. This last group prevailed, and in 1777 a new constitution was adopted, forming the Republic of Vermont. Citing boundary arguments and land claim disputes, the Continental Congress rebuffed the independent republic's request for statehood. Not until 1791 (following a $30,000 land claim settlement awarded to New York) was Vermont finally admitted as the fourteenth state.

Vermont's constitution was the first one to prohibit slavery. It was also the first to establish universal manhood suffrage, overriding the practice of requiring that a man own property or have a specific income level to vote. The constitution was adopted at a meeting held in a Windsor tavern on July 8, 1777, the same day word arrived that British General John Burgoyne and his forces had invaded the Champlain Valley.

Today you can visit the **Constitution House,** the building where the first constitution of the "free and independent State of Vermont" was accepted. A tavern until 1848, it was later turned into shops and quarters for small manufacturing. Still later it was converted into a tenement house, and in 1914 it was moved from its original site to its present location. An official Vermont Historic Site, the former tavern is today a museum housing early Vermont furnishings and artifacts.

You can learn about Windsor's second claim to fame — site of the rebirth of the machine tool industry — by paying a visit to the **American Precision Museum,** located in a formidable brick building originally constructed in 1846 as an armory for the Robbins, Kendall & Lawrence Company. A work force of more than 150 laborers and skilled mechanics produced rifles here when the company was at its peak in the mid-1800s. After the Civil War a cotton mill was established, and sewing machines were manufactured in the building later in the nineteenth century. More recent occupants have included the Windsor Electric Light Company and the Central Vermont Public Service Company. In 1966 the build-

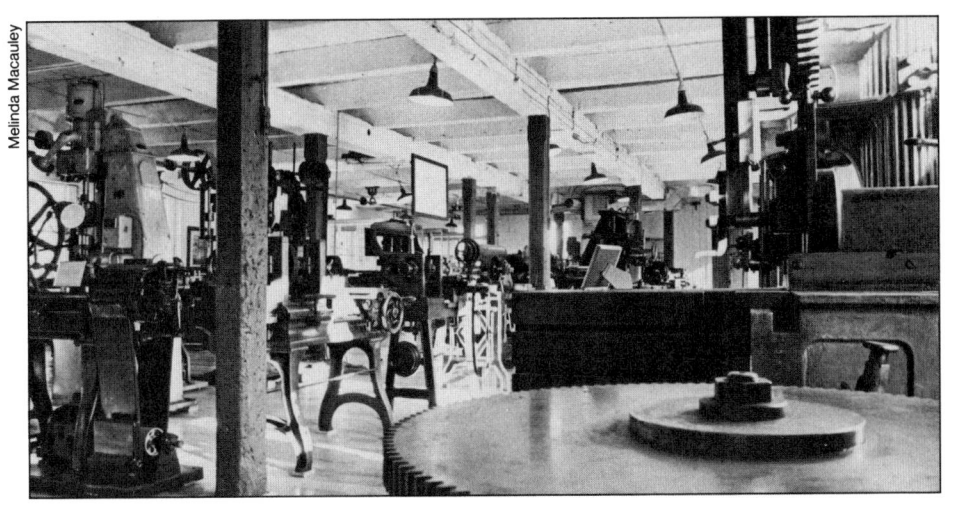

The American Precision Museum's glistening collection is appropriately housed in an 1846 structure built of handmade brick.

ing was acquired by the newly organized American Precision Museum.

Built from handmade bricks and crowned with a slate roof, the museum contains a substantial collection of hand and machine tools, exhibited along with the sewing machines, firearms, knitting machines, and other products they were used to make. White brick walls, polished hardwood floors, and lots of light make an attractive and appropriate backdrop for the abundance of shiny gray, red, black, green, and blue arrangements of wheels, handles, belts, gears, and levers. The equipment on display includes a late nineteenth-century bevel gear grinder, a 1911 multiple-spindle automatic lathe, a 1900 Grindley automatic lathe, and much more.

Since a visit to Windsor is steeped in history, it's fun to continue that theme when it comes time to satisfy your appetite. Consider lunch or dinner at the **Windsor Station Restaurant,** located in the restored Victorian era depot. The decor leans toward brass, natural wood, and velvet, and the menu features veal, beef, seafood, and fowl. California and European wines are served, and the restaurant offers an extensive dessert menu.

Allow plenty of time before leaving Windsor for a stop at the **Vermont State Craft Center,** located in Windsor House, a restored nineteenth-century New England Greek revival hotel. Here you can admire and purchase exquisite pieces created by more than 250 Vermont craftspeople. The juried collection includes fabric arts, many different styles of pottery, leather, pewter, jewelry, baskets, furniture, toys, prints, blown and stained glass, wood, sculpture, and more. The main gallery is filled with pieces that run the gamut from inexpensive paper-craft earrings and necklaces to an antique reproduction wooden jewelry box, from decorative wooden cows and mallards to handcrafted wooden pitchforks.

Upstairs a broad interior balcony connects several specialty areas. One room is set aside as a boutique for wearable crafts. Another is furnished as an early Vermont bedroom, which gives you an opportunity to see the high-quality beds, cupboards, and other pieces in a room setting. A gallery devoted to the work of regional artists opens onto a balcony overlooking Main Street.

If you enjoy working with your hands, you may want to plan your visit to coincide with one of the center's special single-session workshops or lecture/demonstrations. Topics change frequently, but typical offerings include Photography for Beginners, Upholstered Furniture: From the Frame Up, Off Loom Weaving on Hoops, Let's Make a Melon Basket, and The Art of Dry Florals. Inquire about future programs by writing to the Vermont State Craft Center at Windsor House, P.O. Box 1777, Windsor, VT 05089.

Finish your day in Windsor with a brief sidetrip into New Hampshire via the longest covered bridge in the world. Built in 1866 and designated a National Historic Engineering Landmark in 1970, this lovely bridge spans the Connecticut River, connecting Windsor, Vermont, to Cornish, New Hampshire. Cornish is the home of the **Saint-Gaudens National Historic Site,** where you can visit the house and studios in which the artist lived and worked. You can also explore the extensive grounds, which are peppered with gardens and pieces of the artist's work.

One of America's greatest sculptors, Augustus Saint-Gaudens, spent his summers here from 1885

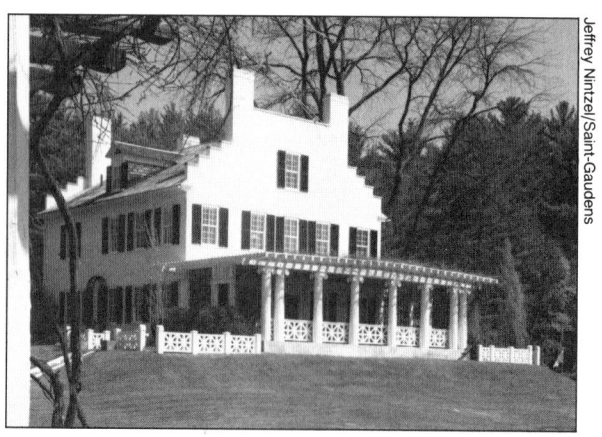

Augustus Saint-Gaudens instructed architects remodeling his long-time home to "make the house smile." They did.

to 1897 before moving in year-round in 1900. He completed nearly 150 sculptures during his lifetime, and his work can be seen in parks, cemeteries, cathedrals, and many other settings in cities including Edinburgh, Paris, New York, Boston, and Washington, D.C.

Your visit begins with a half-hour tour of the artist's house, Aspet, built as a tavern in 1799 to serve travelers on an intended stagecoach road. Today the building is furnished with period pieces, although only some originally belonged to the artist and his family.

When Saint-Gaudens first saw the house in Cornish ten years later, he found it bleak and uninviting. As the story goes, he rented it anyway because he was working on a statue of Abraham Lincoln for a park in Chicago and his friend, Charles Beaman, who owned the house, assured him that the lean, native Yankees would supply him with lots of "Lincoln-shaped" men. Throughout the years that followed, he and his wife remodeled the former tavern (he asked his architects to "make the house smile") and lavished great attention on the grounds, constructing pools, fountains, and even a bowling green. The Saint-Gaudens served as the focal point of a community of about forty artists that continued in Cornish until the mid-1920s.

After the house tour you're free to visit the other buildings and the grounds independently. You'll come upon reproduction bronze reliefs and copies of some of Saint-Gaudens's most famous works. Please note that some parts of the site are wheelchair accessible, while others are not. There is a lovely two-and-a-half-mile trail to hike if you wish. Concerts, mostly chamber music, are held Sunday afternoons in the Little Studio during most of the summer. Feel free to bring along a picnic lunch to enjoy on the grounds before the performance.

The Saint-Gaudens served as the focal point of a community of about forty artists that continued in Cornish until the mid-1920s.

ACCESS

WINDSOR. Traveling north on I-91, take exit 8 to Route 5 north (Main Street) in Windsor. Traveling south on I-91, take exit 9 to Route 5 south (Main Street).

CONSTITUTION HOUSE. Directions: Located on Main Street just north of the Vermont State Craft Center (below). **Season:** Late May to mid-October. **Admission:** Charged. **Telephone:** (802) 674-6628.

AMERICAN PRECISION MUSEUM. Directions: Located at 196 Main Street (Route 5), just south of the Vermont

State Craft Center. **Season:** Late May through October. **Admission:** Charged. **Telephone:** (802) 674-5781.

WINDSOR STATION RESTAURANT. Directions: Located on Depot Avenue, which intersects Route 5 (Main Street) in the center of Windsor. **Season:** Year-round. **Admission:** Free. **Telephone:** (802) 674-2052.

VERMONT STATE CRAFT CENTER. Directions: Located in the Windsor House on Main Street in the center of Windsor. **Season:** Year-round. **Admission:** Free. **Telephone:** (802) 674-6729.

SAINT-GAUDENS NATIONAL HISTORIC SITE. Directions: Located in Cornish, New Hampshire. From Windsor, take the covered bridge to Cornish. Immediately after crossing the bridge turn left and continue 2½ miles on Route 12A north to site entrance, on the right. **Season:** Last weekend in May through October 30. **Admission:** Charged. **Telephone:** (603) 675-2175. **Notes:** Parts of site are handicapped accessible. The covered bridge has been scheduled for extensive repairs. If it is closed, take Route 5 south from Windsor toward Ascutney. Turn left on Route 12. Cross the river, turn left, and continue north on Route 12A to the site.

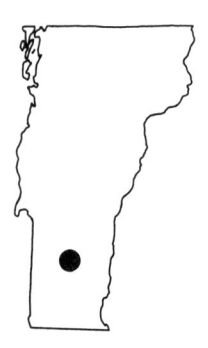

Weston

Pass an unhurried day wandering in and out of cozy shops where the proprietors take special pride in local goods ranging from fudge to firkins. Learn about a tiny rural town's traditions at an eighteenth-century tavern, now organized as a museum. Round out your visit with lunch or dinner and a performance at the Green Mountain State's oldest professional summer theater. Picture-perfect Weston, with a year-round population of about six hundred, is a friendly, accessible country town. Parking is easy, and once you've dispensed with your car, you can walk from one spot to another, enjoying the glorious scenery, a big draw in itself.

If you have extra time, work in a sidetrip to New England's largest winery, a presidential homestead, or a woodland pond, all within an hour of, and in the same direction from, Weston. And should you want to make an extended stay in this part of the Vermont countryside, consider learning a new skill or refining an old one at a residential crafts school located on a former farm.

Let's begin by exploring Weston. Built in 1797, the **Farrar–Mansur House,** located steps away from the village green, is now a historical museum. It is filled with Weston family heirlooms, including a pair of handmade "courting gloves" presented to a young Mansur by his mother on the occasion of his twenty-first birthday. Perhaps the same young man owned the beaver top hat stowed away in its own leather hatbox complete with lock. Designed to serve as a home as well as an inn, the building was a stagecoach stop. Although it did not provide overnight accommodations, Farrar Tavern served refreshments to weary travelers. You'll see the small bar and the two separate rooms — one for ladies and one for gents — where travelers rested and refreshed themselves. The L-shaped kitchen contains all sorts of intriguing equipment, from cherry pitter to wooden corn sheller to old tin coffee roaster, from rat trap to carpet stretcher to lard squeezer.

Upstairs you'll visit the ballroom, which served at different times in its history as courtroom, town meeting room, church, and theater. The adjacent attic space is stuffed to the gills with old toys and textiles, as well as shoemaking, weaving, and spinning equipment. There's also a good collection of guns and swords, carried by local Vermont men in the American Revolution, the War of 1812, and the Civil War, along with their powder horns, knapsacks, canteens, and bayonets.

The ballroom in the Farrar Tavern (now the Farrar–Mansur House) served as the first theater for the **Weston Playhouse**. The roots of the playhouse extend back into the early 1800s, when the local singing society and amateur orchestra decided to undertake dramatic performances along with their musical endeavors. Different performing spaces followed the tavern, and in 1912 the actors formally organized themselves into the Weston Dramatic Club. With the help of a local benefactor, the Congregational Church on the Weston village green, just steps away from the Farrar–Mansur House, was renovated to serve as a theater in 1936, the year the current Weston Playhouse was founded. With its Greek revival portico, stately white columns, and an upstairs lobby opening on a balcony with views of the West River and Mill Pond Waterfalls, the former church, seating nearly three hundred, is well suited as the home of the oldest professional summer theater in Vermont.

A recent year's line-up is typical of the fare produced by the playhouse: *Biloxi Blues, Pippin, I'll Be Back Before Midnight, Chicago, Evita, Oklahoma!,* and *Murder at the Vicarage.* Plan to have a preshow

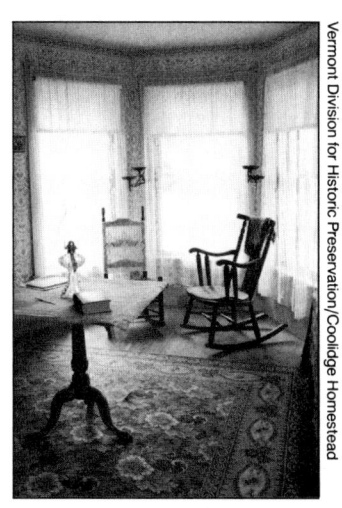

John Coolidge administered the Presidential Oath of Office to his son, Calvin, in this room on August 3, 1923.

lunch or dinner in the English pub ambiance of **Downstairs at the Playhouse.** Lunch features pasta specials, hamburgers, and sandwiches such as The Playhouse Melt — a toasted and buttered English muffin covered with cream cheese, onions, tomatoes, and ham, the whole of it served "under a bubbling blanket of cheddar cheese." For dinner, think about the lobster pie baked with shallots and mushrooms in white wine and cream, topped with puff pastry. Desserts include Swiss nut torte and strawberries Romanoff. After the evening performances, the restaurant is transformed into a cabaret, offering even more entertainment.

There are lots of intriguing shops within walking distance of the village green. Craftspeople at the **Weston Bowl Mill** produce large quantities of woodenware year-round. It's fun to look into the rooms where workers operate jigsaws, lathes, and drills, producing all sorts of useful and decorative items. The store is lined with shelves of lazy Susans, lapdesks, rolling pins, and salad bowls. Firkins and footstools cover the floor, and the air is filled with the scent of fresh sawdust. Bird feeders hang above the stacks of candleholders, silverware trays, birch plates (finished and unfinished), and bins of novelty items that vary from wooden mushrooms to wooden nickels. There's a factory annex, too, where you can purchase woodenware "seconds" at reduced prices.

Taken in 1902, this photo shows the Weston Bowl Mill and its staff "the way they were."

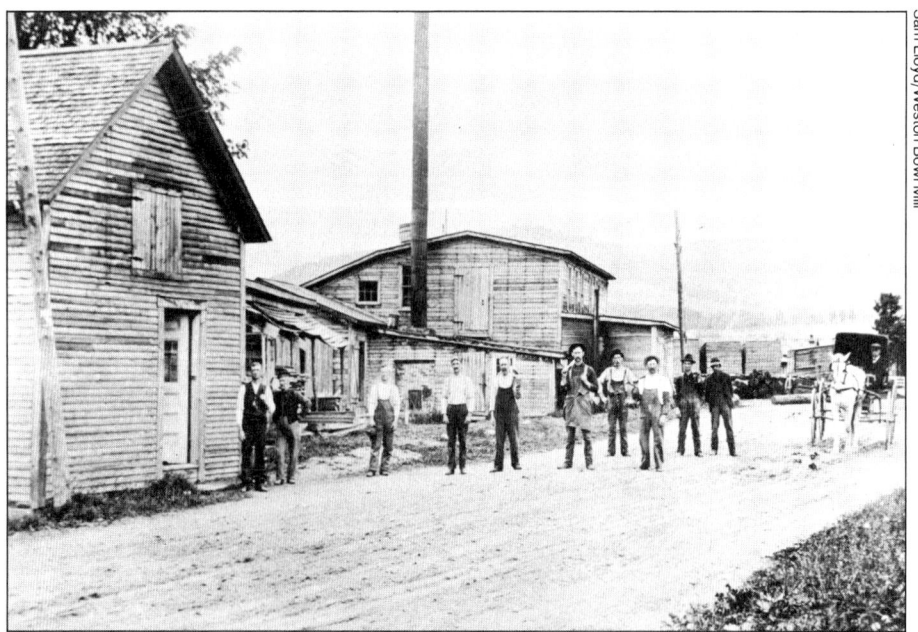

Looking for a sinfully delicious snack? The sweet smell of fresh chocolate tells you that you've come to the right place as you enter the **Weston Fudge Shop.** Most of the candy sold here is made on the premises in full view of customers. There are many flavors, from chocolate mint and maple walnut to Grand Marnier and amaretto. There's also fabulous raspberry-almond bark and an outstanding butter crunch. And the shop makes and sells its own ice cream. Treat yourself to a sundae, cone, or shake, or opt for a rich hot chocolate on a chilly day.

It's fun to shop at the **Vermont Country Store,** which overflows with New England food specialties and country-style clothing and kitchenware. Calico is sold by the yard just as it was a hundred years ago, and of course there's that all-important curved-glass candy case resplendent with old-time confections.

When you've finished prowling through these and the many other shops in town, you might want to make a sidetrip off Route 100 to the **Hapgood Pond Recreation Area** in the Green Mountain National Forest, where you can cool off with a swim on a hot day or take a hike in the woods when the foliage is at its peak. The seven-acre pond is edged by a sandy beach on the west side. The area has forty picnic sites with tables and grills, as well as twenty-eight camping sites should you wish to stay overnight. You can launch your canoe or small boat (no motors, please), and fishing is permitted (with a valid state license) except in the swimming area. A nature trail just a little under a mile long winds around the pond from the north edge to the east side. You'll have many views of the water during the half-hour hike that takes you over a bridge and across a dam. Benches are provided for rests along the way.

Returning to Route 100 north, it's just a short ride to the **Joseph Cerniglia Winery,** the region's newest and largest wine-making facility. The first wine was bottled here in the fall of 1986. The Cerniglia Winery is the only New England producer of premium apple wines. Unlike other apple wines, those produced here are varietals rather than blends. That means only one type of apple goes into each wine. The Granny Smith is dry and crisp, while the McIntosh resembles a good Chablis, and the Red Delicious yields a sweet table wine much like a sauterne. But we're getting ahead of ourselves. Tour first; taste later.

As you tour the winery, you'll be introduced to

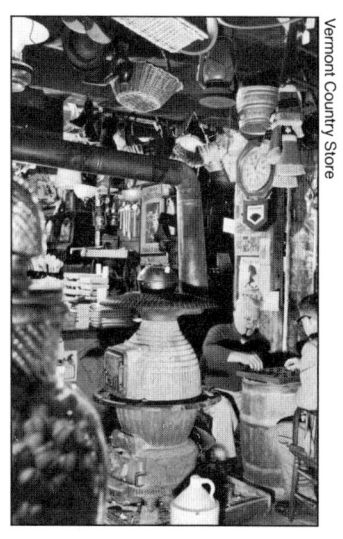

Time didn't really stop at the Vermont Country Store in the 1950s when this picture was taken; it just feels that way when you step inside.

the processes involved in transforming millions of apples into premium wines, wine coolers, champagne, and hard cider. The fruit goes first through the washer and grinder and then to the hydraulic press. After that it is stored in huge fermentation tanks until it is ready for filtering. The operation wraps up with bottling, corking, and labeling. There are no short cuts when it comes to producing Cerniglia wines. They go through the same painstaking processes used to produce premium grape wines.

Now it's time to step up to the long wine-tasting bar to sample the product and "talk wine" with a knowledgeable staff member. You'll be given five or six different wines to taste. Common crackers are offered between wines to cleanse the palate. The wines are, naturally, for sale. And don't forget the wine coolers (this is the only New England winery that produces them), which contain twenty percent fruit juice and five percent alcohol and are as refreshing a treat as you can imagine on a hot summer day. Choose from apple-apple, raspberry, orange, and twist of lemon. The hard cider is just about perfect when the leaves are shuffling underfoot and there's a bright fire burning in the showroom fireplace. Wine accessories and local crafts are offered for sale, along with Vermont cheeses, jams, and other local culinary treats. Put together a lunch or snack to savor at one of the picnic tables on the winery grounds overlooking the Black River.

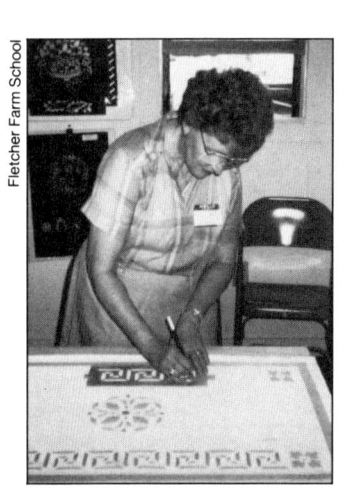

Course offerings at Ludlow's Fletcher Farm School for the Arts and Crafts range from stenciling to weaving and Ukrainian egg decorating.

Extend your stay in the Green Mountains by enrolling in a course at the **Fletcher Farm School for the Arts and Crafts** in Ludlow, operated by the nonprofit Society of Vermont Craftsmen. Conducted by experienced craftspeople with lengthy credentials, the workshops and classes are held in a group of eighteenth-century farm buildings. The course catalog lists about sixty introductory and advanced workshops, which last from a weekend to five days. Workshops in the decorative arts cover subjects such as theorem painting, wall stenciling, and Norwegian rosemaling. In fiber arts, you can study beginning four-harness loom weaving, spinning and natural dyeing, and Scandinavian weaving techniques, to name just a few. Furniture refinishing, ornamental carving, and decoy carving are typical of the woodworking courses, while pieced quilting and crewel embroidery are among the needlework options. Workshops also focus on subjects as diverse as basketry, music, herbal arts, early American bandbox construction, and Ukrainian egg decorating.

Classes are usually held from 9 A.M. to noon,

and again from 1 to 4:30 P.M. Studios remain open until 9 P.M. The farm offers comfortable accommodations, single and double rooms with shared bathrooms, for those wishing to live "on campus." Family-style meals are served (you'll know it's time for dinner when the cowbell rings), and in the evening fellow students often play chamber music. If you think you might like to enroll in a workshop, write to the Fletcher Farm School for the Arts and Crafts, R.R. 1, Box 1041, Ludlow, VT 05149, for a detailed course catalog.

The **Calvin Coolidge Homestead** in Plymouth Notch, a short distance from Ludlow, is preserved just as it was at 2:47 on the muggy morning of August 3, 1923, when Calvin Coolidge was sworn in as the country's thirtieth president by his father, a Vermont notary public. You can also visit Coolidge's birthplace, where his family lived before moving into the homestead in 1876. It contains furnishings actually used by the family, including the bed in which the future president was born in 1872.

Across the street from the homestead, the **Wilder Barn** is filled with tools for splitting shingles, shelling corn, and harnessing dog power. It contains butter churns, cheese presses, and a foot-powered milking machine. Period vehicles include the shiny yellow coach that delivered mail along the Woodstock–Reading route, as well as an RFD mail sled for winter deliveries. Also visit the **Plymouth Cheese Corporation,** the factory operated by the president's family, where cheese is still made today. You can watch the small production plant in operation and sample the cheese or purchase other New England foods such as honey, baked beans, relishes, pickles, and canned hash. If you require immediate sustenance, head over to the **Wilder House,** the home of Coolidge's mother, where you can purchase ice cream and sandwiches.

The Calvin Coolidge Homestead in Plymouth Notch is preserved just as it was on August 3, 1923, when Coolidge was sworn in as the country's thirtieth president.

ACCESS

WESTON. Follow I-91 to exit 1, Brattleboro. Follow signs to Route 30. Take Route 30 west to Route 100 north. Follow Route 100 north to Weston.

LUDLOW AND PLYMOUTH. Follow directions to Weston. Continue north on Route 100 to Ludlow and farther north to Plymouth.

FARRAR–MANSUR HOUSE. Directions: Located on Route 100, by the village green in Weston. **Season:** Late May through mid-October. **Admission:** Charged. **Telephone:** None.

WESTON PLAYHOUSE. Directions: Located on Route 100 in Weston. **Season:** July through early September. **Admission:** Charged. **Telephone:** (802) 824-5288.

DOWNSTAIRS AT THE PLAYHOUSE. Directions: Located in the Weston Playhouse building. **Season:** July through early September. **Admission:** Free. **Telephone:** (802) 824-5288.

WESTON BOWL MILL AND ANNEX. Directions: Located on Route 100 in Weston. **Season:** Year-round. **Admission:** Free. **Telephone:** (802) 824-6219.

WESTON FUDGE SHOP. Directions: Located on Route 100 in Weston. **Season:** Year-round. **Admission:** Free. **Telephone:** (802) 824-3014.

VERMONT COUNTRY STORE. Directions: Located on Route 100 in Weston. **Season:** Year-round. **Admission:** Free. **Telephone:** (802) 824-3184.

HAPGOOD POND RECREATION AREA. Directions: From Weston, follow Route 11 west about 5 miles to Hapgood Pond. **Season:** Early May through late September. **Admission:** Free. **Telephone:** None.

JOSEPH CERNIGLIA WINERY. Directions: From Weston, follow Route 100 north to Ludlow. Turn right at the intersection with Route 103 then right on Winery road, at sign to winery. **Season:** Year-round. **Admission:** Free. **Telephone:** (802) 226-7575. **Note:** Winery is handicapped accessible.

FLETCHER FARM SCHOOL FOR THE ARTS AND CRAFTS. Directions: Follow Route 100 north to Ludlow. Turn left at the intersection with Route 103. Continue west to Fletcher Farm School, on the left. **Season:** Late July through August. **Admission:** Tuition, room, and board fees. **Telephone:** (802) 228-8770.

CALVIN COOLIDGE HOMESTEAD. Directions: Follow Route 100 north from Ludlow toward Plymouth. Turn right on Route 101A and follow signs to homestead. **Season:** Mid-May through mid-October. **Admission:** Charged. **Telephone:** (802) 828-3226.

For further information or restaurant and lodging suggestions, contact the Ludlow Chamber of Commerce, Depot and Bridge Street, Ludlow, VT 05149. Telephone: (802) 228-5318.

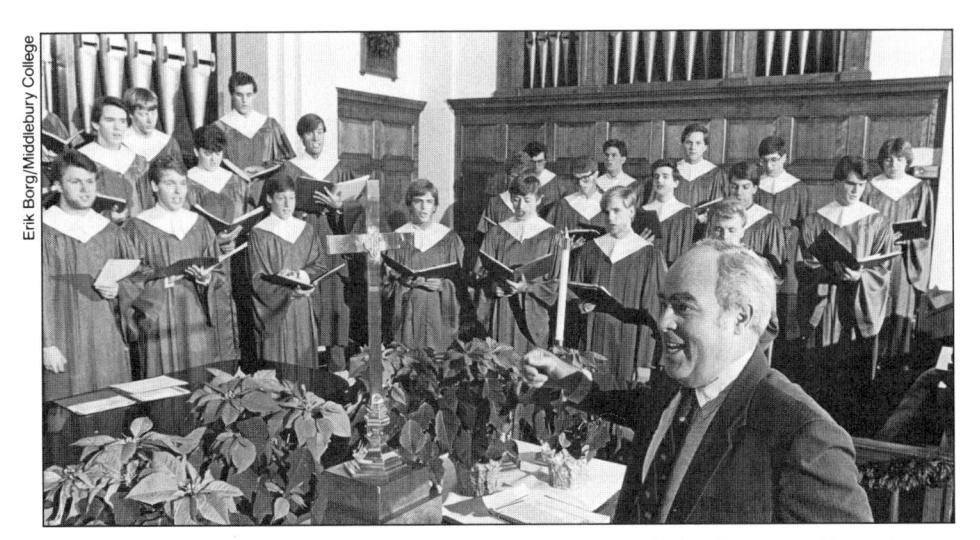

Both college ensembles and visiting artists contribute to the Middlebury College Concert Series.

Middlebury

In 1761 the King of England chartered three towns to be built in a forest of hemlock and pine bordering a running river in what is now Addison County, Vermont. Two of them, New Haven and Salisbury, were named for the Connecticut towns that the new towns' settlers left behind. The third, the one in the middle, was logically enough named Middlebury. An inauspicious start, perhaps, but Middlebury has done well for itself. A thriving college town in a pastoral setting, with the Green Mountains to the east and the Adirondacks to the west, Middlebury is charming and alive. Settle in for one day or several. Play a round of golf or do some skiing. Attend a concert or art exhibit. Prowl in the specialty shops or pick berries in a sun-drenched field, just as you did when you were a child. There's plenty to do, yet the pace is relaxed and informal, and the crowds are conspicuously absent much of the year.

The town is the home of prestigious Middlebury College, and visitors can take advantage of the many cultural events the college sponsors. The **Middlebury College Concert Series** provides a varied program of first-rate performances throughout the academic year. A typical schedule might list appearances by the Vermont Symphony Orchestra, the Boston Viol Consort, the Meliora String Quartet, and the New York Vocal Arts Ensemble. The college publishes a seasonal schedule of events, which also lists other campus activities such as lectures, films, the-

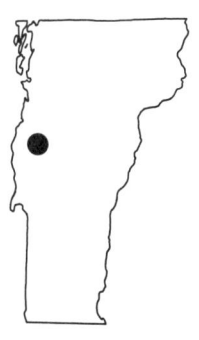

For a favorite grandchild, you might want to splurge on a whimsical toy like the airplane with a carrot body, string bean propellers, lettuce wings, and tomato wheels.

ater and dance performances, and athletic events. Something is happening nearly every evening.

The college opens some of its athletic facilities to visitors, in particular the attractive eighteen-hole **Ralph Myhre Golf Course of Middlebury College.** Snack bar and pro shop are located in the Alumni Conference Center overlooking the course. Joggers enjoy the 3.5 km John "Red" Kelly '31 Trail, which loops around the golf course. In winter the trail is lighted for night cross-country skiing. At the **Middlebury College Snow Bowl,** also open to the public, two double chair lifts and two pomalifts serve thirteen trails and slopes, accommodating both novice and expert downhill skiers.

Be sure to allow time to wander through downtown, particularly the Frog Hollow section, where small factories produced nails, pails, wooden products, and guns at a fever pitch in the early 1800s. The first marble in the state was quarried, cut, and polished here, too, with power supplied by the rushing waterfalls of Otter Creek. Today the old factory buildings house an interesting assortment of shops, most notably the **Vermont State Craft Center at Frog Hollow.**

The center bills itself as the leading advocate of crafts in the state. A nonprofit organization dedicated to encouraging excellence in Vermont crafts and to providing first-rate craft instruction, the center markets the work of more than two hundred Vermonters, most of them full-time craftspeople. Many have organized cottage industries where they employ others to help produce their wares, giving the center far-reaching economic importance.

Situated overlooking Otter Creek Falls, the bright, airy gallery is chock-full of wonderful handmade pieces. We fell in love with a hooked rug doormat showing an elephant surrounded by fruits. Also available were stenciled place mats and woven table runners, baskets, prints, many styles of pottery, pewter plates and bowls, a marble chess set, and elegant red oak beach chairs with handwoven slings. For a favorite grandchild, you might want to splurge on a whimsical toy like the airplane with a carrot body, string bean propellers, lettuce wings, and tomato wheels. Well, you have to see it to appreciate it.

If you enjoy working with your hands, plan your visit to Middlebury around one of the workshops offered by the center. There are many one- and three-day courses, some intended for those with previous experience and others open to both beginners and more advanced craftspeople. Past workshops include Stone Carving, Painting, Absolute Photography, Appalachian Egg and Melon Baskets, and Hand-quilting. Write to Vermont State Craft Center at Frog Hollow, Middlebury, VT 05753, for a schedule of classes.

Nancie Dunn, who served as the center's gallery director for ten years, has recently opened her own shop just a few feet away. **Sweet Cecily,** named after a favorite herb and a special daughter, does not feature Vermont crafts but instead concentrates on folk art and contemporary crafts from all over the country. This means Western folk art, Mexican pieces, Victoriana, and much more. "The pieces run from the sublime to the ridiculous," explains Nancie. "There are items for $2 and others for $500, but all are wonderful, and I've met all the people who make them." With its doorstep garden and whimsical decorating touches (some pieces are displayed on painted oak chairs hung on the wall as shelves), the shop is fun to explore.

Used book and record fans should drop in at **The Alley Beat,** located a couple of steps up from street level across from the craft center. You can hear the waterfall in the background as you browse through shelves and tables of paperbacks and hardcovers that will likely include works by Dickens and Dostoyevsky along with contemporary tales by such writers as Colleen McCullough, Sidney Sheldon, and John Le Carré. The record selection includes classical and jazz. Well lit, with a couple of chairs to rest on and soft music in the background, this small shop is a pleasant place to pick up some vacation reading.

The **Otter Creek Café & Bakery** is a great place to satisfy your appetite, whether you're looking for an afternoon snack or a well-prepared full-course meal. Dine indoors in the bottom of an old stone mill or out on the wooden deck, where tables topped with purple-and-white umbrellas overlook Otter Creek. Both lunch and dinner are served. The day we visited, the menu listed cream of leek and garlic soup; hot duck pâté in puff pastry; and scaloppini of veal with watercress, white wine, and cream, along with crêpes, omelettes, and several fish dishes. The restaurant is fully licensed.

Instead, you might choose to order a generous sandwich to go, made up on delicious homemade bread in the bakery. Settle down to eat and relax at one of the picnic tables right on the bank of the

One- and three-day workshops for both beginning and experienced craftspeople complement the exhibits at the Vermont State Craft Center at Frog Hollow.

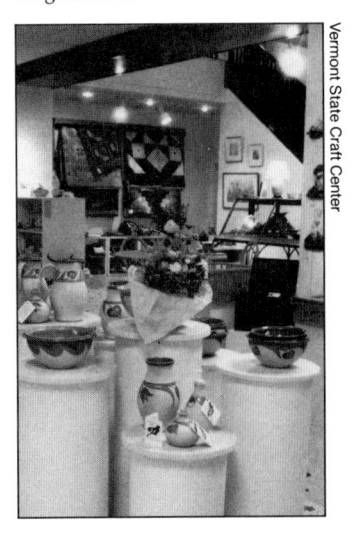

creek. Wherever you eat, don't ignore dessert. Well worth the calories, selections run the gamut from homey oatmeal-raspberry squares to chocolate-strawberry torte with Grand Marnier. For those in-between times when hunger strikes, consider cinnamon-raisin honey buns, cranberry-bran muffins, or perhaps a couple of English scones.

To get a sense of Middlebury's history, take a tour of the **Sheldon Museum,** a five-minute walk from Frog Hollow. A three-story brick Federal style house with six black marble fireplaces, the museum contains furniture, clocks, pewter, toys, textiles, tools, musical instruments, and other accoutrements of daily life in nineteenth-century Vermont. The collection was started in 1875 by Henry L. Sheldon, who was born on a nearby farm in 1821. His self-assigned mission was to preserve every detail of his beloved Vermont heritage. Many of the items in the collection are accompanied by brief notes Henry penned describing the article and its origins.

Your visit takes the form of a forty-five-minute guided tour, beginning in the front parlor where a special exhibit is displayed each year. You'll learn that Henry Sheldon first became acquainted with the building when it served as a boarding house. He rented a room and eventually purchased the building, which he immediately incorporated as a museum. A versatile fellow, he bought, sold, and repaired pianos, worked on the railroad and in a bookstore, bound books, and served as town clerk. He kept detailed diaries and labeled everything that came his way, determined as he was to show how people lived in his day.

You'll see the borning room, where children came into the world and the elderly prepared to depart from it. You'll visit the kitchen and see a table set with Henry's pewter. Pointing to the cup plates, your guide will explain that it was once thought good manners to pour the beverage into the saucer to cool, place the cup on the cup plate, then drink the liquid directly from the saucer.

Exploring the house from top to bottom, you'll come upon all sorts of items, from a standup secretary of bird's-eye maple and mahogany veneer to tiny early bifocal glasses, from a Middlebury College study chair complete with rockers and arm desk to a collection of bonnets and hatboxes. There are musical instruments, too, from drums to a collection of wooden flutes. And don't be shocked by the stuffed cat, permanently at rest on Henry's bed. A woman in nearby Cornwall gave it to Henry to preserve more

Henry L. Sheldon, whose private collection became the Sheldon Museum, took it upon himself to "preserve every detail of his beloved Vermont heritage."

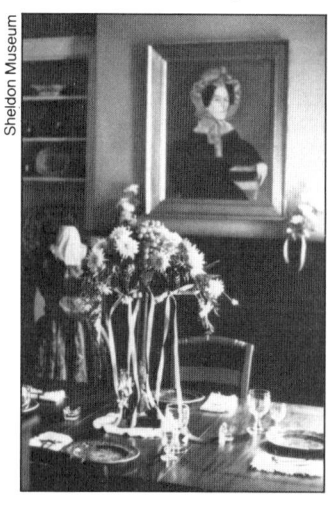

than a hundred years ago, and, as we've indicated, Henry wasn't one to throw anything out. That's why his museum is such a pleasure to explore.

Elsewhere in Middlebury, a few miles from the center of town, you can visit the **University of Vermont Morgan Horse Farm** and learn all about the history of this remarkable breed of equine. Born in Springfield, Massachusetts, in 1789 — the same year that George Washington became president — a slight colt named Figure was destined to become the progenitor of the first light-horse breed in America. His owner, schoolmaster Justin Morgan, brought him to Vermont in 1791 in search of a better life. Morgan wanted to sell Figure (who was later renamed Justin Morgan) but couldn't find a buyer because of the colt's diminutive size. But Figure proved himself fast, versatile, and strong over the next thirty years, and it was through his three colts — Sherman, Bulrush, and Woodbury — that America's first breed of horse was founded.

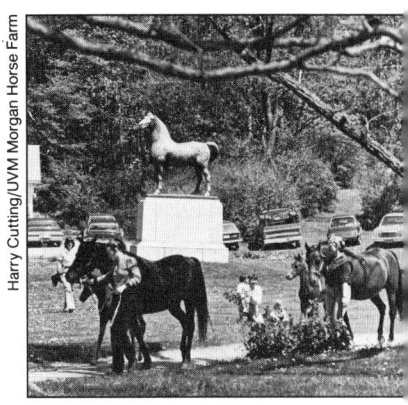

The small but versatile Morgan horse — America's first breed — was bred right here in Middlebury, where the University of Vermont today operates the Morgan Horse Farm.

The Morgan Horse Farm was established in 1907 to perpetuate the Morgan breed. Morgan horses have continued to grow in popularity over the years, serving as cavalry mounts, ranch horses out West, farm horses, and riding horses. Approximately seventy registered stallions, mares, and foals live at the farm, whose horses have been shipped as far afield as Sweden, China, Peru, and Israel.

Inside the ornate Victorian barn you'll see displays of harnesses and horseshoes, ribbons, trophies, photographs, and other Morgan memorabilia. A slide show introduces the farm and its residents, with an explanation of selective breeding and farm management. Next your guide will lead you on a tour of the barn and grounds. The air is heavy with the scent of leather, horse, and hay as you peer into spacious stalls and stroke a warm muzzle here and there to make the acquaintance of some of these handsome animals. More than twenty foals are born here each year, and you may well see some of the youngsters kicking up their heels in the rolling fields. After the tour, pull out a picnic to enjoy on the grounds of the horse farm, possibly one of the most glorious spots in all Vermont.

Just north of Middlebury in New Haven, you can spend an hour picking fresh fruit at **Granstrom's Fruit Farm**. The fields are rimmed by woods and distant mountains, and the only house in sight is the farmhouse. Strawberries, grown in neat rows mulched with straw, come into their own in mid-June. Raspberries, which require less bending, are

The air is heavy with the scent of leather, horse, and hay as you peer into spacious stalls and stroke a warm muzzle here and there.

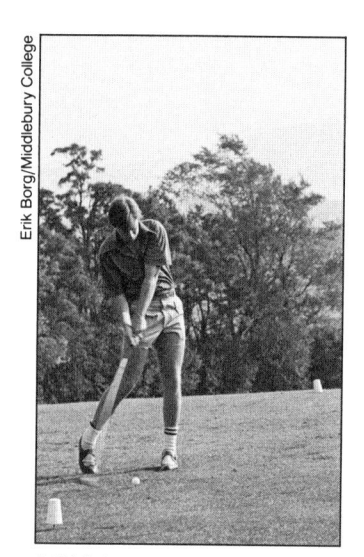

Middlebury College's Ralph Myhre Golf Course is open to the public.

ready by the middle of July. Baskets and boxes are supplied, and you pay by the pound. Should you pass through in the fall, you can pick apples instead.

ACCESS

MIDDLEBURY. Follow I-91 north to Bellows Falls/Route 103 exit. Take Route 103 west to Route 7. Follow Route 7 north to Middlebury. Turn left after The Middlebury Inn to get on Route 30 (Main Street).

MIDDLEBURY COLLEGE CONCERT SERIES. Directions: Performances are held in Mead Chapel and Wright Theater, on the Middlebury College campus. **Season:** September through April. **Admission:** Charged. **Telephone:** (802) 388-3711, ext. 5697. **Note:** For a schedule, write to Middlebury College Concert Series, Johnson Memorial Building, Middlebury, VT 05753; also request the Middlebury College calendar of events.

RALPH MYHRE GOLF COURSE OF MIDDLEBURY COLLEGE. Directions: Entrance located on South Main Street (Route 30), south of the Paris Fletcher Field House. **Season:** April through November, depending on weather. **Admission:** Charged. **Telephone:** (802) 388-3711, ext. 5125.

MIDDLEBURY COLLEGE SNOW BOWL. Directions: Located 15 miles from the main campus. Traveling north on Route 7, turn right on Route 125. Continue east on Route 125 to the Snow Bowl. **Season:** December to April. **Admission:** Charged; senior discount. **Telephone:** (802) 388-4356.

VERMONT STATE CRAFT CENTER AT FROG HOLLOW. Directions: Located on Mill Street in the Frog Hollow area, one-half block off Main Street (Route 30). **Season:** Year-round. **Admission:** Free. **Telephone:** (802) 388-3177.

SWEET CECILY. Directions: Located in Frog Hollow, a few steps from the Vermont State Craft Center. **Season:** Year-round. **Admission:** Free. **Telephone:** (802) 388-3353.

THE ALLEY BEAT. Directions: Located in Frog Hollow in the long brick building across from the Vermont State Craft Center. **Season:** Year-round. **Admission:** Free. **Telephone:** None.

OTTER CREEK CAFÉ & BAKERY. Directions: Located in the bottom of the Frog Hollow Mill building on Frog Hollow Road, off Main Street (Route 30). **Season:** Year-round. **Admission:** Free. **Telephone:** (802) 388-7342.

SHELDON MUSEUM. Directions: Located at 1 Park Street in the center of town. **Season:** Year-round; limited hours November through May. **Admission:** Charged; senior discount. **Telephone:** (802) 388-2117.

UNIVERSITY OF VERMONT MORGAN HORSE

FARM. Directions: Leaving Middlebury, head west on Route 125. Just beyond the small rotary, turn right onto Route 23, which is Weybridge Street. Follow signs to farm, about 2½ miles. **Season:** May 1 through October 31. **Admission:** Charged. **Telephone:** (802) 388-2011.

GRANSTROM'S FRUIT FARM. Directions: Take Route 7 north from Middlebury for 3 miles. Turn right on River Road, following signs to farm. **Season:** Mid-June through early August; September to November. **Admission:** Free. **Telephone:** (802) 388-3912.

For further information or restaurant and lodging suggestions, contact the Information Center, 35 Court Street, Middlebury, VT 05753. Telephone: (802) 388-7579.

Shelburne

People from all over the world flock to the **Shelburne Museum.** Founded in 1947 by Mr. and Mrs. J. Watson Webb, an extremely wealthy couple, to "show the craftsmanship and ingenuity of our forefathers," the museum contains the finest collection of folk art in the country. An impassioned collector who began acquiring Americana seriously in 1913, before just about anyone else, Electra Havemeyer Webb was determined to share her things with the public. After World War II, she and her husband began the museum with just one building on eight acres of land. But as Electra's passion for collecting continued to grow, they bought additional land and moved other structures to the site, including the 892-ton steamboat *Ticonderoga*.

Neither a restoration nor a reconstructed village, the museum calls itself a "collection of collections." More than forty buildings are spread out over the meticulously landscaped grounds. The range and depth of the exhibits housed here make the Shelburne Museum perfect for travelers who are able and willing to take the time to truly appreciate them.

Because of the size of the museum, you may want to purchase an economical two-day pass. If your time is limited, you may be best off studying the museum guide carefully and targeting collections related to your most pressing interests, be they fine arts, antique toys, decorative arts, antique furniture, or nineteenth-century commercial life.

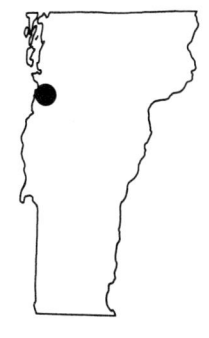

However you choose to organize your visit, the **Passumpsic Round Barn** is a good place to get your bearings. Here you can view a slide show detailing the history of the museum and a large-scale model of the grounds and buildings, which makes it easy to figure out how to get to the places where you wish to spend your time.

The exhibits are spread out over forty-five acres, but you can drastically reduce the amount of walking by taking advantage of the free jitney (a sort of land-bound barge with seats, pulled by a tractor), which makes a regular loop through the grounds. Board and reboard as often as you like. Jitney or not, it is almost impossible to absorb everything the museum has to offer in a single day.

Outdoors enthusiasts may want to take a look at the North American game paintings in the Beach Gallery and the big-game trophies in the Beach Hunting Lodge, which also houses Northwest Coast and Plains Indian artifacts, as well as boats used by the Indians in hunting expeditions. If you are enchanted by decorative arts and textiles, don't miss the intricate stump-work embroideries in the Prentis House and the overwhelming assemblage of crewel work, samplers, hooked rugs, quilts, coverlets, and hand-painted wallpaper in the Hat and Fragrance Unit. The Dorset House contains more than a thousand early decoys, Audubon game-bird prints, fowling pieces, and miniature and decorative carvings. The Toy Shop is chock-full of dolls, wooden toys, puppets, penny banks, and music boxes, several of which are in working order. The museum also includes a wonderful 1920 vintage merry-go-round, which operates daily.

Some of the structures at the museum were designed to house specific collections, such as the semicircular Circus Building, which contains a 525-foot scale model of a circus parade. Carved and decorated performers from all over the world form the procession, which boasts acrobats and tumblers, men on stilts, and dozens of clowns, along with seals, elephants, bears, dogs, and magnificent circus wagons drawn by teams of horses.

Other buildings are exhibits in their own right, quite apart from the wonderful treasures they display. Some of these include the Shelburne Railroad Station, a fine example of Victorian architecture; the Colchester Reef Lighthouse; and, of course, the *Ticonderoga*, the last vertical-beam passenger and freight side-wheel steamer intact in the United States. While you're at the railroad station, take a walk through the private railroad car complete with luxurious sofas and beds and a built-in bathtub. What a way to travel!

In addition to textiles, decoys, cigar store and carousel figures, weather vanes, trade signs, primi-

If you are enchanted by decorative arts and textiles, don't miss the intricate stump-work embroideries.

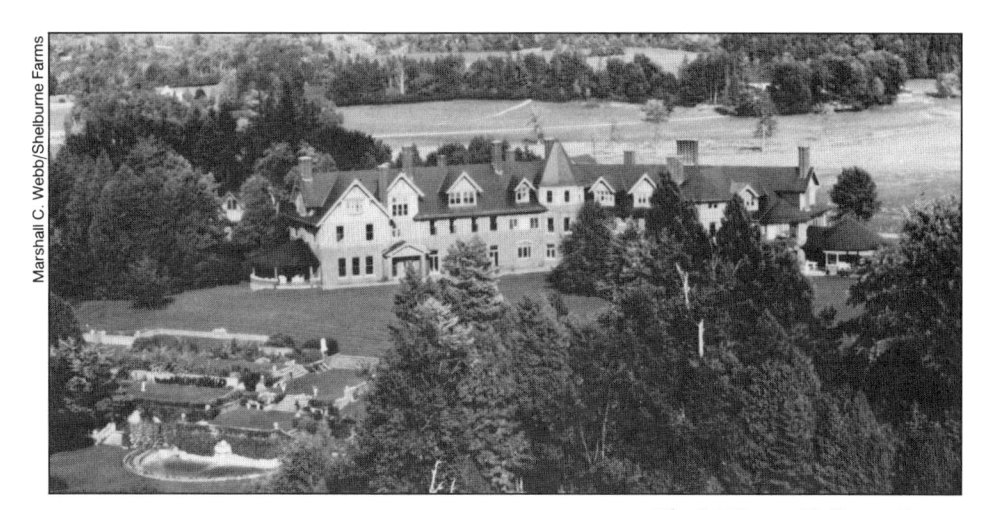

The 1,000-acre Shelburne Farms served as a summer residence for wealthy New Yorkers beginning in the 1880s.

tive drawings and paintings, and painted furniture, the Webbs acquired many fine European pieces. The Electra Havemeyer Webb Memorial Building houses old master and impressionist paintings, as well as Degas bronzes and re-created furnished rooms from the Webbs' New York City apartment, which give a sense of the good life Electra led.

For a different perspective on the way the rich managed their lives, take a guided tour of **Shelburne Farms,** a thousand-acre agricultural estate created in the l880s as a summer residence by Dr. William Seward and his wife, Lila Vanderbilt Webb. Your visit begins in the Visitor Center, where you will see a brief slide show, "For Those with Vision," describing the history of the farm. Shelburne Farms was designed by noted landscape architect Frederick Law Olmsted (who also designed New York's Central Park) and Gifford Pinchot, a founder of the American conservation movement. As many as fifteen thousand trees and shrubs were planted on the farm in its heyday. Farm buildings borrow from several architectural styles, including Old English, Queen Anne revival, and Romanesque.

After the slide show, board a bus and travel along a three-and-a-half-mile winding road to Lake Champlain. Actually the lake is only a mile from the Visitor Center, but Olmsted created this approach, and even had many of the hills built, to give a sense of endless land.

You'll leave the bus for a walk through the **Coach Barn.** The architect who designed it was involved primarily in designing railroad stations, and that influence is readily evident. The brick barn surrounds a courtyard, and the walls are of a slightly

Shelburne Farms was designed by noted landscape architect Frederick Law Olmsted (who also designed New York's Central Park) and Gifford Pinchot, a founder of the American conservation movement.

different height on each side. There are eyebrow windows on one side, Tudor style on another. Some of the stalls remain in use, and the original woodwork is intact in the harness room.

Reboard the bus and head for **Shelburne House,** where the family summered. Built in the Queen Anne revival style with turreted towers, it recreates the feeling of an old manor house filled with lords and ladies. The restored garden, with its semicircular lily pond, wanders downhill toward the lake, accented by brick walls, stone steps, and statuary. The plantings were chosen to create the feeling of an impressionist painting. Concerts are held several times each summer on the south porch of the house, and visitors are welcome to bring along picnics to enjoy on the broad lawn overlooking the lake before the performance. Inquire about the schedule.

Shelburne House also operates as an inn, and if you love the countryside, you may want to pass a night or two here, relaxing in elegant surroundings that contain many of the original furnishings that came from Lila Webb's family. The inn has twenty-four bedrooms and a lovely dining room featuring regional country food. Even if you do not stay at the inn, you might like to have breakfast or dinner here. Reservations are required for both meals.

Board the bus again, this time to ride to the dairy barn, built in the 1930s as a commercial venture to keep the farm from going broke in the aftermath of the Depression. A herd of brown Swiss cows was assembled at that time, and the same line occupies the barn today, providing fresh milk to make fine "Farmhouse Cheddar" (which means that all the milk used to produce the cheese comes from cows on the property). More than 190 cows live here, but half are too young for milking. A good cow produces twenty thousand pounds of milk a year. You can rub some warm, moist noses in the open barn, which is filled with the clunky ring of cowbells. You can also watch the cheese-making process through the large observation window or step into the milking parlor, where four cows are accommodated at one time.

Then it's back on the bus and off to the last stop, the huge farm barn. With its two-acre courtyard and stalls for eighty horses, this used to be the center of activity at Shelburne Farms. The lower floors are made of red limestone, and the upper are mostly shingled. The central portion of the barn, five stories high, is topped by a tower. The turrets and roofs are coated in copper now green with age. At the turn of the century, when Shelburne Farms provided work for thirty house servants and more than a hundred farm hands, the barn housed a bakery, blacksmith, and wheelwright. Although in disrepair, it is still a most impressive structure and evokes poignant images of a long-gone era.

The tour ends back at the Visitor Center, where you can sample the cheeses produced at the farm and take a look in the **Farm Store,** which stocks the makings of a fine picnic, complete with bread and wine. If you have time, you can take a stroll on the walking trail, which winds from the visitor center to the south side of the farm barn and up Lone Tree Hill before looping back to the start. Nearly one hundred species of birds have been sighted in the vicinity of the trail, so you may want to bring your binoculars.

A couple of miles south of Shelburne along Route 7 is Charlotte. At the **Vermont Wildflower Farm** you can take a leisurely walk through six acres of wildflowers, grown in natural settings. The daily "bloom report" is posted at the start of the path, which winds through open fields and shaded woodlands. Several benches along the route provide places for you to sit and enjoy the surroundings. Be sure to pause on the viewing platform over the marsh to listen to the cacophony of bird and bullfrog noises, to watch the delicate blue "darning needles" dash between the cattails, and to discover the clusters of delicate forget-me-nots.

More than 250 species of wildflowers are grown here, and you'll be given a garden guide appropriate to the time of year you visit. The guide briefly describes the origin and use of the plants, hinting at the ancient herbal and romantic legends associated with many of them. Major flower species are described in greater detail on sturdy Plexiglas placques positioned along the path. St. Johnswort, just a weed to many of us, turns out to have been named for St. John the Baptist. In medieval Europe it was used to ward off witches, devils, and the evil eye. When crushed into an ointment, its blossoms became "balm of the warrior's wound," and it served as a major medicinal plant on the medieval battlefield.

In the farm shop you can purchase wildflower seeds for your own garden. Each packet is displayed beneath a color photograph of the plant in bloom so you know what you're buying. If you have always longed for a field of wildflowers like those painted by the French impressionists, you can start to make your dream into a reality by choosing an annual or perennial wildflower mix designed specifically for your part of the country and your garden conditions.

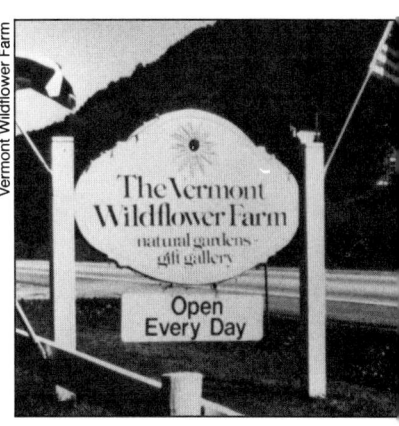

More than 250 species of wildflowers are grown on the Vermont Wildflower Farm. Visitors receive a garden guide appropriate to the time of year.

There are mixes for shady areas, partial shade, and full sun, as well as for moist and dry areas. The shop also stocks all sorts of gifts with a flower theme.

Did you ever go berry picking as a child? Does the idea of plucking sun-warmed fruit fresh from the plant sound appealing? At the **Charlotte Berry Farm** you can gather strawberries, raspberries, or blueberries, depending on the time of summer you visit. When the weather is hot, you'd do well to time your visit early in the morning before the sun gets fierce; otherwise bring along a hat. Just follow the berry signs out to the field, where insects buzz and birds sing. An attendant will direct you to a row for picking. Containers are provided, and you'll pay for your berries by the pound. A couple of tables are available, and you're welcome to bring along a picnic if you like.

Continuing a little farther south along Route 7, you'll see signs to **Mount Philo State Park,** where you can enjoy lovely views of the Lake Champlain Valley from the summit of the 980-foot mountain. A network of about fifty trails, some of them very steep, crisscrosses the park, yet you don't need to walk more than a few yards from the parking lot to relish a panorama of farms and fields. Picnic tables are situated to take advantage of the views, some in the shade and some in the sun. Hawks are frequent visitors here, and golden eagles make an appearance several times a year. The park has sixteen tent sites and three lean-tos, along with hot showers. Reservations are recommended for weekends.

Another way to savor the scenery is to take a ride on Lake Champlain aboard the **Charlotte–Essex Ferry**. This small blue-and-white ferry serves not primarily as a tourist boat but as a means of convenient transportation between Vermont and neighboring New York State. If you intend to stay in Vermont and just want to go along for the ride, buy an inexpensive foot passenger ticket. The crossing takes about twenty minutes each way, but allow an hour for the round trip because of the time spent loading and unloading cars. Hot dogs and ice cream cones are sold at the ferry landing.

ACCESS

SHELBURNE. Take I-89 to exit 13. Follow I-189 west to Route 7. Continue south on Route 7 to Shelburne.

CHARLOTTE. Continue south on Route 7 from Shelburne about 3 miles.

SHELBURNE MUSEUM. Directions: Take I-89 to exit 13.

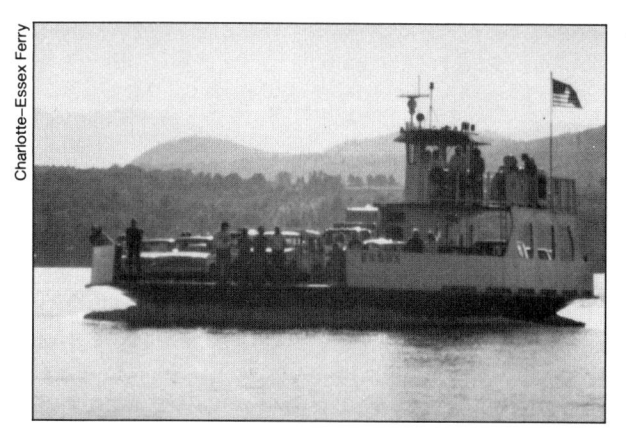

You can go along just for the ride on the Charlotte–Essex Ferry, which shuttles passengers across Lake Champlain between Vermont and New York State.

Follow I-189 west to Route 7. Go south on Route 7 through the town of Shelburne to the museum entrance on your right. **Season:** Mid-May through mid-October. **Admission:** Charged. **Telephone:** (802) 985-3344. **Note:** A few wheelchairs are available at the ticket booth. Several buildings have ramped entrances, including the *Ticonderoga*, the cafeteria, and the rest rooms in the railroad station.

SHELBURNE FARMS. Directions: Follow I-189 west to Route 7. Continue south 3 miles and turn right on Bay Road. Shelburne Farms is at the end of the road. **Season:** Tours from June 1 through mid-October; shop open year-round. **Admission:** Charged. **Telephone:** (802) 985-8686.

SHELBURNE HOUSE. Directions: Located at Shelburne Farms. **Season:** June 1 though mid-October. **Admission:** European and MAP offered. **Telephone:** (802) 985-8686.

VERMONT WILDFLOWER FARM. Directions: Located on Route 7 in Charlotte. **Season:** May through mid-October. **Admission:** Free. **Telephone:** (802) 425-3500.

CHARLOTTE BERRY FARM. Directions: Located on Route 7 in Charlotte. **Season:** Late June through late August. **Admission:** Free; purchase what you pick. **Telephone:** (802) 425-3652.

MOUNT PHILO STATE PARK. Directions: Continue south on Route 7 about 3 miles past Vermont Wildflower Farm. Turn left at flashing light on unmarked road at sign for Mount Philo State Park. **Season:** Last weekend in May through Columbus Day. **Admission:** Charged. **Telephone:** (802) 425-2390.

CHARLOTTE–ESSEX FERRY. Directions: From Burlington, follow Route 7 to Route F-5 in Charlotte. Turn right and continue 3 miles to ferry. **Season:** Varies; usually April through December, depending on ice. **Admission:** Charged. **Telephone:** (802) 864-9804.

For further information or restaurant and lodging suggestions, contact the Shelburne Business Association, Box 383, Shelburne, VT 05482. Telephone: (802) 986-2296.

VERMONT / 143

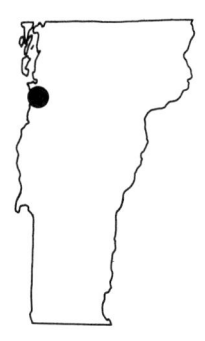

Burlington

Snuggled up close to the Canadian border in the northwest corner of Vermont, Burlington combines the cultural attractions of a college town with the natural attraction of lovely Lake Champlain. Here you can watch the manufacture of two unusual Vermont products (chocolate and cheesecake) in the morning, explore the lake or a first-class art museum in the afternoon, and attend a concert or play — or even a professional minor league baseball game — in the evening. A bit off the beaten path (many people head only to well-known Shelburne just a few miles south), Burlington combines the cultural attributes of a college town with several unusual discoveries. (What's a chocolate factory doing in northern Vermont?) Although it is a city, Burlington is manageable in size, making the trip from one attraction to the next — on foot or in a car — a relaxed one.

Start out by satisfying your sweet tooth at **Champlain Chocolate,** where you can take a factory tour and sample the product. Your guide will introduce the history of chocolate, using a large map to point out the parts of the world where cocoa beans grow, giving the delicious confection its start. She'll show you where and how the ingredients are combined to make fine candy, and explain the way the temperature table and foil wrapping machine work. During the twenty-minute tour you're likely to see candy makers at work shaping, dipping, and decorating chocolates. This is hands-down the best smelling factory tour you're ever likely to take. Tours are offered on Tuesday, Wednesday, and Thursday, and you need to call the day before to reserve a place.

Back in the small showroom overlooking the production areas, you can purchase some of the sinfully delicious stuff. Champlain Chocolate specializes in American truffles, great golf ball–size handmade chocolates with delicate ganache centers. They come in many varieties, including mandarin orange, Grand Marnier, raspberry, and bourbon pecan. Also produced is a line called Chocolates of Vermont. Made in hand-carved molds with Vermont motifs such as the maple leaf or pine tree, they are individually wrapped in brightly colored foil.

Only the freshest, top-quality ingredients are used in these chocolates, and the candy-making process is extremely labor-intensive. No wonder the price is so hefty. Here at the factory, however, you can treat yourself to reduced-price seconds. They may

Champlain Chocolate specializes in American truffles, great golf ball–size handmade chocolates with delicate ganache centers.

Sampling the goods is only part of the fun at the Cheese Outlet, where tours and retail bargains also are available.

not be quite as pretty as their perfect cousins, but they taste just as splendid.

Just across the street from the chocolate factory you can do some serious sampling at the **Cheese Outlet,** northern New England's largest wine and cheese warehouse. Bargain hunters will have a field day here. As general manager Steve Lidle notes, "We take problems off people's hands. To make it as an outlet, you have to offer some outrageously good buys. We purchase monstrous amounts of things, so we get them really inexpensively. That means we can give big discounts, sometimes as much as seventy-five percent off." One example is the forty thousand pounds of Swiss cheese Lidle recently purchased for peanuts from an importer who had overordered and needed to unload the stuff.

On a typical day, you'll find more than seventy varieties of cheese from which to choose, along with nearly as many wines, which also are purchased in bulk and priced to move. Also available to tempt you are specialty foods including the most popular seller, honeycup mustard packaged in plastic containers. It sells here at less than half the price you'd pay in fancier stores, where it comes in pretty little jars. You can even taste a bit before deciding to purchase, just as you can with any of the cheeses.

The folks here don't make cheese, but they do produce thirty-two thousand quiche puffs and four thousand Vermont Velvet cheesecakes each week, more than any other factory in New England. Tours of the plant, which adjoins the salesroom, are offered every weekday morning. One product is produced each day, either the cheesecake or the quiche, depending on the orders that need to be filled. These items are sold to cruise ships, airlines, hotels, even jails. You'll see where the products are mixed, baked,

On a typical day, you'll find more than seventy varieties of cheese from which to choose, along with nearly as many wines.

VERMONT / 145

and cooled. And of course you'll get to taste the end result. You might want to purchase some cheesecake cookies from the outlet to munch on your way out.

Appetite satisfied, go on to explore some of Burlington's cultural attractions. The city is the home of the University of Vermont, which welcomes visitors to its **Fleming Museum,** home of four permanent collections: fifteenth- to nineteenth-century European paintings and sculpture; eighteenth- and nineteenth-century American paintings, furniture, costumes, and decorative arts; Southeast Asian and Chinese art; and Asian and ancient Egyptian art. Special exhibits and a lively schedule of lectures, concerts, and other events complement the collections. The museum shop stocks prints, books, note cards, glassware, and other gifts.

Just a five-minute walk from the museum, professional actors gather each summer at the university's Royall Tyler Theatre to present the **Champlain Shakespeare Festival,** which has delighted audiences for more than thirty seasons. The theater can accommodate nearly three hundred people, and seating is on three sides of the thrust stage, which means that no seat is more than six rows away from the actors. It's fun to arrive an hour early and sip soft drinks or a glass of beer or wine on the piazza outside the theater. In addition, most performances are preceded by another show, perhaps a classical dance or guitar solo.

If you visit Burlington during the school year, telephone the theater for information on the four productions staged annually by University of Vermont theater students. All productions are open to the public.

Music lovers might want to look into performances of the **Craftsbury Chamber Players,** who

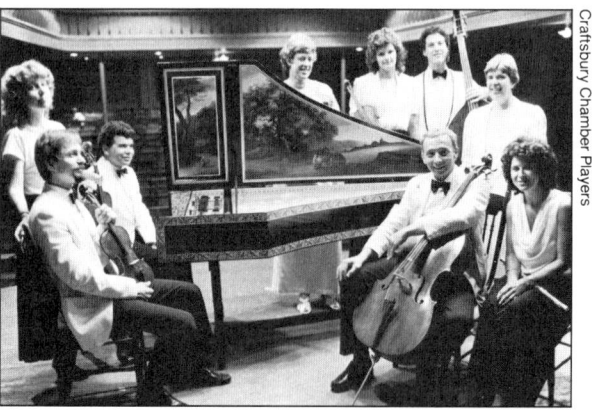

The Craftsbury Chamber Players have treated northern Vermont to their special music since 1964.

have treated northern Vermont to lovely chamber music since 1964. Weekly summer concerts are presented at St. Paul's Cathedral in Burlington. A recent schedule included an evening of Vivaldi and Debussy and a second combining Schubert songs, a Corigliano sonata, and a Brahms piano trio. Tickets can be purchased in advance or at the door.

Burlington's **Battery Park** also comes alive with music each week during the summer. Bring along a lawn chair or blanket and watch the sun set over Lake Champlain as you enjoy the outdoor early evening concerts. The fare includes classical, folk, blues, country, and some rock, performed by both nationally known and local musicians. Also once a week throughout the summer Ben & Jerry's presents a free, feature-length outdoor movie.

Speaking of which, ice cream fans will want to stop in at the original **Ben & Jerry's,** located in a former gas station right in downtown Burlington, where the ever-popular black-and-white cow on a background of blue sky and green grass is omnipresent, even painted on the upright piano. The music tends toward the loud, but the atmosphere is pleasant. Have a fresh fruit sundae made with Ben & Jerry's famous chunk-filled flavors or lemonade squeezed right before your eyes.

You can also purchase Ben & Jerry's ice creams from the pushcart that works the **Church Street Marketplace,** an outdoor pedestrian mall in the downtown area. The mall is lined with shops, restaurants, and several outdoor cafés for fair-weather dining and excellent people watching.

For quite a different type of entertainment, attend a **Vermont Reds** baseball game. A minor league team associated with the Cincinnati Reds, Vermont's only professional team is a perennial contender in the eight-team Eastern League. Games are played at the university's Centennial Field.

We've still only begun to scratch the surface of the entertainment options in Burlington. The **Flynn Theatre** is the scene of performances that run the gamut from the Duck's Breath Mystery Theater to the Finnish National Symphony Orchestra to the Kingston Trio. The box office also sells tickets to dozens of other area events.

Last but by no means least is Burlington's natural attribute, Lake Champlain. To appreciate and enjoy the lake fully, take a shoreline cruise aboard the *Spirit of Ethan Allen.* During the one-and-a-half-hour narrated trip you'll hear stories about French explorer Samuel de Champlain and his Algonquin

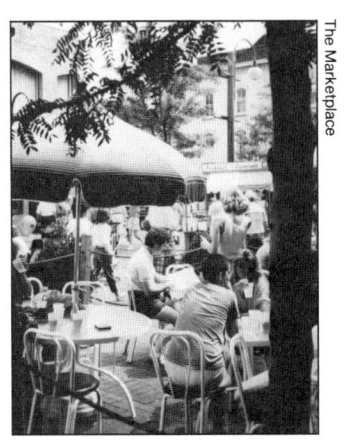

The Marketplace

For shopping, dining, and people watching, you'll want to pay a visit to downtown Burlington's Church Street Marketplace.

In 1984, seventy passengers aboard the Spirit of Ethan Allen *excursion boat spotted "Champ," the legendary serpent of Lake Champlain.*

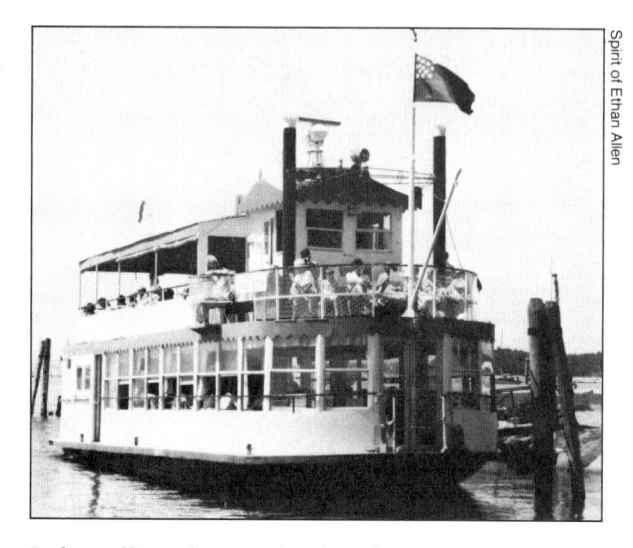

Spirit of Ethan Allen

Indian allies, along with tales of Ethan Allen and his Green Mountain Boys. In July 1984 seventy passengers aboard this ship sighted "Champ," the legendary serpent who lives in the lake. Maybe you too will catch a glimpse. Lake Champlain's largest excursion vessel, the *Ethan Allen,* has an open upper deck and a fully enclosed heated lower deck. She sails rain or shine. Two-hour sunset cruises and dinner cruises are offered on alternate evenings, and three-hour moonlight dance cruises are offered on Saturday nights.

ACCESS

BURLINGTON. Follow I-89 to Burlington.

CHAMPLAIN CHOCOLATE. Directions: From I-89, take I-189 west to Route 7. Traveling north on Route 7 toward Burlington, turn left on Flynn Avenue, then immediately right on Pine Street. The factory store is at 431 Pine Street. **Season:** Year-round; midweek tours, call ahead. **Admission:** Free. **Telephone:** (802) 864-1808.

CHEESE OUTLET. Directions: Located diagonally across from Champlain Chocolate at 400 Pine Street. **Season:** Year-round. **Admission:** Free. **Telephone:** (802) 863-3968.

FLEMING MUSEUM. Directions: Take I-89 to exit 14W. Follow Route 2 west to the University of Vermont campus. Museum is located on Colchester Avenue on the campus. **Season:** Year-round. **Admission:** Free. **Telephone:** (802) 656-2090.

CHAMPLAIN SHAKESPEARE FESTIVAL. Directions: Located at the Royall Tyler Theatre on the University of Vermont campus. **Season:** July through mid-August. **Ad-**

mission: Charged; senior discount. **Telephone:** (802) 656-2094. **Note:** Theater is handicapped accessible.

CRAFTSBURY CHAMBER PLAYERS. Directions: Performances at St. Paul's Cathedral in Burlington, located on St. Paul's Street in downtown. **Season:** Mid-July through late August. **Admission:** Charged; senior discount. **Telephone:** (802) 586-9644. **Note:** Concerts are handicapped accessible.

BATTERY PARK SUMMER CONCERTS. Directions: Presented at Battery Park, between Lake Street and Battery Street, which borders Lake Champlain. **Season:** Late June through mid-August. **Admission:** Free. **Telephone:** (802) 656-2095.

BEN & JERRY'S. Directions: Traveling west on Route 2 (Main Street), go right on South Winooski Avenue. Continue three blocks to Cherry Street. Located at 169 Cherry Street. **Season:** Year-round. **Admission:** Free. **Telephone:** (802) 862-9620.

CHURCH STREET MARKETPLACE. Directions: Located in the center of downtown Burlington on Church Street, between Main Street (Route 2) and Pearl Street. **Season:** Year-round. **Admission:** Free. **Telephone:** (802) 863-1648.

VERMONT REDS. Directions: Games played at Centennial Field, off East Avenue on the University of Vermont campus. **Season:** Mid-April through August. **Admission:** Charged. **Telephone:** (802) 862-6662.

FLYNN THEATRE. Directions: Located at 153 Main Street (Route 2). **Season:** Year-round. **Admission:** Charged. **Telephone:** (802) 863-5966.

SPIRIT OF ETHAN ALLEN. **Directions:** Departures from Perkins Pier in Burlington. Take I-89 to exit 14W. Take Route 2 west about 2 miles, following signs to ferries. Perkins Pier is located at the foot of Maple Street, one block south of where the ferries dock. **Season:** Late May through mid-October. **Admission:** Charged. **Telephone:** (802) 862-9685. **Note:** Handicapped accessible.

For further information or restaurant and lodging suggestions, contact the Lake Champlain Regional Chamber of Commerce, Box 443, 209 Battery Street, Burlington, VT 05402. Telephone: (802) 862-9685.

MAINE

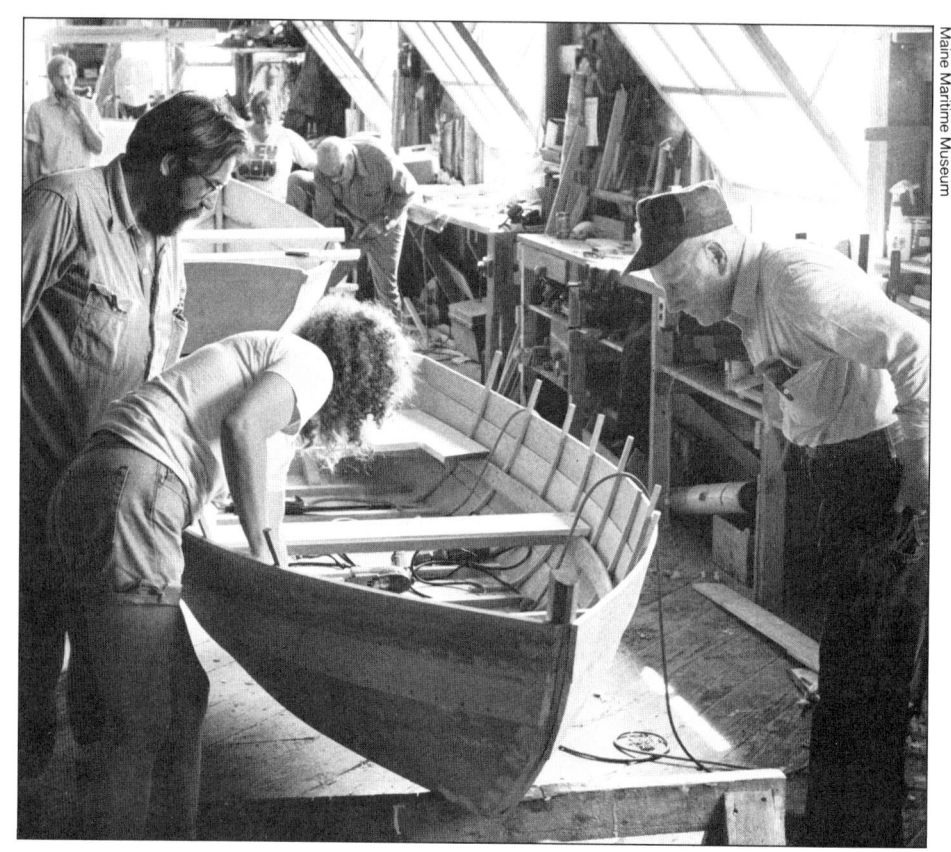

Wooden boat construction remains a living tradition at the Percy and Small Shipyard, part of the Maine Maritime Museum in Bath. Wooden sailing vessels are built here, as well as smaller, handcrafted dories like these.

Freeport

Freeport is synonymous with **L.L. Bean,** the giant outdoor equipment and clothing mail-order business, whose retail store is open 24 hours a day, 365 days a year. The friendly tone is set right in the parking lot, where you'll notice picnic tables and a sign that reads, "Is your dog hot? Fresh water available here." The L.L. Bean store is almost an obligatory stop for anyone driving along the southern Maine coast. What most visitors don't realize, however, is that there is much more to do here than just shop.

You may want to enroll in the **L.L. Bean Fly Fishing Schools.** The Introductory School offers personal instruction in basic fly casting, fly presentation, and fishing, enabling even those who have never fished before to advance quickly. Based in Freeport, the school is organized in three-day sessions. Each session covers fly fishing and philosophy, tackle choice and balance, useful knots, basic fly casting, fly presentation and fishing, natural foods and how to imitate them, fly tying, fishing apparel, safety, and conservation. Participants are videotaped so that they can watch themselves in action, while an instructor offers advice for improving technique. A basic fly-fishing outfit is provided to each student as part of the course.

The Intermediate School is designed for fishermen who have already mastered the skills presented in the introductory course. Each session lasts four days, with two-thirds of the instructional time spent on the water. Sessions are held in the Grand Lake Stream area of Maine. Subjects taught include entomology, reading water, knots, wading techniques, canoe fishing, and advanced casting techniques. You will also be instructed on how to cast and fish dries, wets, nymphs, streamers, and salmon and bass flies.

These courses fill up very quickly. Reservations are accepted as early as January for the following season (mid-April through July). Of course, if you decide you'd like to attend at the last moment, it's worth calling to find out if anyone has canceled.

For a new twist in evening entertainment, attend one of the free **L.L. Bean clinics** offered throughout the year at the retail store in Freeport and at the L.L. Bean Casco Street Conference Center less than a mile away. Typical programs cover topics such as Trout Cookery: Stream to Table; Spring Birding in Maine; Summer Day Hikes in Maine; and Freshwater Trolling: Gear and Strategy. Clinics begin at 7:30 P.M., last one or one and a half hours, and are held several times each week. Most involve a combination of slide show, lecture, and demonstration.

If you have never canoed and would like to learn, you might want to enroll in the **L.L. Bean Paddling Lesson,** a two-hour introductory session held on the Royal River in Yarmouth and conducted by the L.L. Bean staff. The lesson is intended for beginners, and all equipment is provided. Sessions are offered several times a day on Saturdays in May and June, and advance reservations are required.

The Bean store itself is huge, a veritable department store. The fishing department, which is larger

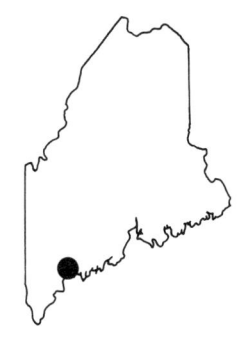

L.L. Bean offers classes in cooking, hiking, fly fishing, and canoeing in addition to serving in its traditional role as a retail outlet.

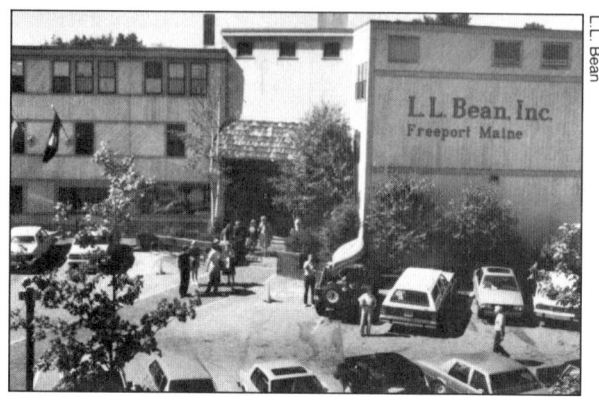

It is interesting to note that of the first hundred pairs of shoes Leon L. Bean sold, ninety were returned when the rubber bottoms separated from the leather uppers.

than your average sporting goods store, is subdivided into sections devoted to spin fishing, fly fishing, and saltwater fishing. There's even an indoor trout pond, located below the freestanding staircase leading from the men's department to the women's department. Landscaped with rocks, greenery, and even its own waterfall, the pond is alive with indigenous Maine brook trout, which can be found throughout the state in freshwater streams, ponds, and lakes, and even in brackish or salt water.

Elsewhere you'll discover a full department of Maine-made products, including pie, cake, and picnic baskets and pottery decorated with blueberries, sheep, fruit, and flowers. Food specialties include canned dandelions, raspberry honey, and sardines from Port Clyde. Bargain hunters should check out the second-floor factory store, where clothing for men, women, and children is peddled at discount prices that often reach fifty percent.

Back in 1912, Leon L. Bean created a new hunting shoe, a lightweight leather-and-rubber design that was destined to become the foundation of a thriving multimillion-dollar business. He began his entrepreneurship by sending a mailing to holders of Maine hunting licenses. It is interesting to note that of the first hundred pairs of shoes he sold, ninety were returned when the rubber bottoms separated from the leather uppers. Bean refunded the money, went back to the drawing board, perfected his product, and started selling like crazy. By 1927 he had added fishing and camping gear to his catalog, and by 1937 sales passed the million-dollar mark. You can still purchase L.L. Bean's Maine hunting shoe, in the store or by mail, along with all sorts of other well-made clothing and equipment.

Freeport, a shopper's paradise, features not only L.L. Bean but also a profusion of factory outlet stores on Main Street and nearby. At the Dansk Factory Outlet you can save up to sixty percent on seconds and discontinued Dansk products — casual dinnerware, teakwood serving pieces, flatware, glassware, and cookware. If your tastes run to the more formal, take a look at the fine china and handcrafted crystal at the Lenox China and Crystal Outlet. Attractive leather shoes and comfortable sandals await at the Bass Shoe Factory Outlet, and tons of shirts and other men's clothing are available at the Hathaway Factory Outlet. The Freeport Outlet contains Londontown (a London Fog outlet store), the Leather Outpost (offering a complete line of Buxton leather goods and accessories), and several other stores. And that's just a sampling. A complete directory to the outlets is posted right outside the main entrance to the L.L. Bean store. All the stores sell discontinued products, seconds, and overstocks priced substantially below retail, and they are all open year-round. Keep them in mind when you start your holiday shopping and feel you need a change of scenery from your local mall.

For a brief respite from the frenetic Freeport shopping pace, ask the folks at **The Wine Cellar** to fix up a handsome picnic that you can take to a restful spot. This tiny shop specializes in wine, cheese, and fancy food items. They also assemble deli sandwiches such as sliced turkey and provolone on a sesame seed roll or dill Havarti with lettuce, tomato, and dressing on a bulky onion roll.

Just a five-minute ride from town, a good place to picnic is the **Mast Landing Sanctuary,** maintained by the Maine Audubon Society. After lunch, take time to explore the nature trails that wind through the 150-acre preserve. Or take your picnic a bit farther afield in the direction of South Freeport. At **Winslow Memorial Park** you can settle down at a table on the broad green lawn overlooking the ocean. There's also a small sandy beach where you can sample the refreshing (to put it mildly) Maine water. Other amenities include a boat launch and offshore island camping (inquire ahead).

South Freeport itself feels a million miles away from Freeport proper. On your way there, you'll pass through an elegant pastoral scene complete with well-kept farmhouses and cows and sheep peacefully grazing in the fields. Then you'll drive down a quiet country road and find yourself at a pleasant dead end overlooking a saltwater inlet. The view is studded with lobster buoys, a pine-covered island, and a cluster of creaking lobster boats bobbing at the

Freeport, a shopper's paradise, features a profusion of factory outlet stores on Main Street and nearby.

dock. Lobsters writhe in the holding trap tied to the dock, as you listen to the squawks of the sea gulls swooping overhead and the splash of water lapping at the shore.

Harraseeket Lunch, a low-slung barn-red building perched on the edge of the inlet, specializes in seafood baskets filled with fried scallops, clams, and the like. The menu also includes steamed clams, boiled lobsters, and clam cakes, along with hamburgers and even turkey sandwiches for those who favor an ocean view but don't have a hankering for seafood. Homemade brownies and whoopie pies are the dessert favorites. There are dining areas indoors and out, as well as take-out service.

It's worth making the sidetrip to South Freeport just for lunch and atmosphere. While you're here, however, take a look inside the chandlery at **South Freeport Marine,** where you can tend to serious nautical needs such as sailboat and deck hardware, navigation and safety gear, paint, and charts. The yard itself rents Rhodes nineteen-foot sailboats and sixteen-foot Privateer outboard motorboats by the half day and full day, offering a perfect way to explore the coves and bays.

If you admire fine woodwork and feel like venturing a bit farther into the rural Maine countryside, we suggest a sidetrip to tiny Bowdoinham, home of **The Decoy Shop.** The shop is actually a factory that manufactures decorative and hunting decoys for shipment all over the world. The unpretentious showroom is lined with rows of finished decoys, unfinished decoys, half models, and gift items made from decoys.

The first decoys made by the company back in the 1930s were working decoys. Their bodies were made from Portuguese cork so they would float and not reflect sunlight, and their bills were carved in Eastern white pine. The Decorative Cork Collection features nonworking decorative copies of those early decoys. The Primitive Collection is modeled after decoys used by the Indians. It includes a sea gull, goose, mallard, swan, and loon, all roughly carved in Canadian white cedar. The Penobscot Bay Collection features large waterfowl carved from solid pine, with the bill and feather details carved by hand. Hand-finished miniature decoys, individually shaped and sanded, also are produced here, along with a line of marine wildlife carvings that includes harbor seals and humpback and beluga whales.

Hobbyists who would rather *make* their folk art than buy it can purchase ready-to-finish, individ-

Each bird crafted at Bowdoinham's The Decoy Shop is completely hand-painted and signed by the artist.

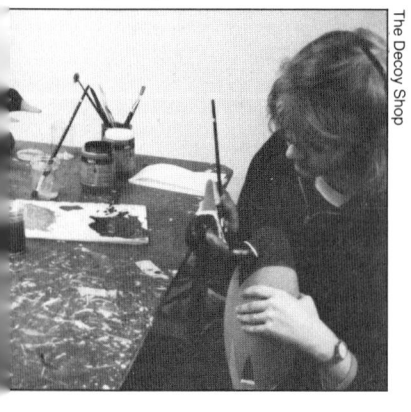

ually shaped and sanded select pine carvings. Unfinished decoys, roughly carved, also are sold in kit form.

If you call ahead, you can tour the factory, filled with racks of bodies and heads awaiting assembly. The smell of sawdust thickens the air as you watch a craftsperson operate the carving machine, which shapes sixteen birds at a time on sixteen different spindles. In the finishing room, the hunting decoys are painted with stencils. The company employs about twenty-five craftspeople, many of whom work at home, to do the hand-carving and hand-painting. Each decoy is slightly different and is signed by the artist. In case you don't make it to Bowdoinham, take a look at the decoys at L.L. Bean, where you'll find birds made at The Decoy Shop.

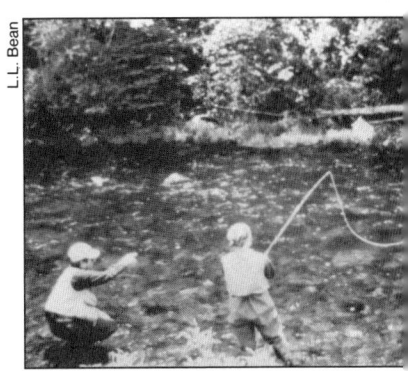

Expert instruction from the L.L. Bean Fly Fishing Schools includes on-site (knee-deep) training.

ACCESS

FREEPORT. Follow I-95 to exit 18. Take Route 1 north into Freeport.

L.L. BEAN. Directions: Located on Route 1 in the center of Freeport. **Season:** Year-round; Fly Fishing Schools operate from mid-April through July. **Admission:** Free. Fee charged for Fly Fishing Schools. **Telephone:** (800) 341-4341.

THE WINE CELLAR. Directions: Follow Route 1 to Mechanic Street in Freeport, at the corner between the Bass and Hathaway outlets. Located at 2 Mechanic Street. **Season:** Year-round. **Admission:** Free. **Telephone:** (207) 865-3404.

MAST LANDING SANCTUARY. Directions: Follow Mechanic Street to Upper Mast Landing Road. Turn left and continue 1 mile to sanctuary. **Season:** Year-round. **Admission:** Free. **Telephone:** None.

WINSLOW MEMORIAL PARK. Directions: From Freeport, follow Route 1 south to South Freeport Road. Turn left on South Freeport Road, then right on Staples Point Road at sign for Winslow Park. **Season:** April through September; weekends only in April. **Admission:** Charged. **Telephone:** (207) 865-4198.

HARRASEEKET LUNCH. Directions: From Freeport, follow Route 1 south to South Freeport Road. Turn left and follow signs. **Season:** Late May through mid-October. **Admission:** Free. **Telephone:** (207) 865-4888.

SOUTH FREEPORT MARINE. Directions: Chandlery is located next to Harraseeket Lunch in South Freeport. Marina is just across the street. **Season:** April through October. **Admission:** Free. **Telephone:** (207) 865-3181.

THE DECOY SHOP. Directions: Follow I-95 north to exit 25. Take Route 125 into Bowdoinham. The shop is located at the lower end of Main Street, just beyond the blinking light at the intersection with Route 24. **Season:** Year-round. **Admission:** Free. **Telephone:** (207) 666-8461. **Note:** Call ahead if you wish to visit the factory.

For further information or restaurant and lodging suggestions, contact the Maine Publicity Bureau, 97 Winthrop Street, Hallowell, ME 04347. Telephone: (207) 289-2423.

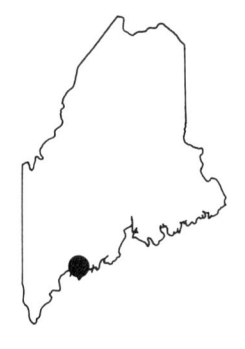

Bath

Nicknamed the "City of Ships," Bath has a long and honorable tradition when it comes to building boats. Great sloops and schooners were produced in the shipyards lining Bath's wharves during the last half of the nineteenth century, making it the fifth busiest seaport in the country. Between 1896 and 1920, forty-one wooden sailing vessels were constructed at the Percy and Small Shipyard, the only American yard still building that kind of boat.

Many shipyards went out of business with the advent of steel ship production in the 1890s, but with the founding of Bath Iron Works (BIW) in 1894 (also still in operation), shipbuilding continued to be an important industry here. Today Bath is a study in contrasts. You might see a four-hundred-foot steel frigate undergoing an overhaul at BIW, while down the road at Percy and Small apprentices learn the craft of traditional wooden boatbuilding.

A visit to Bath centers on the **Maine Maritime Museum,** with indoor and outdoor exhibits in two different parts of the city. You'll probably begin at the ten-acre site of the Percy and Small Shipyard on the banks of the Kennebec River. Here you can roam through restored buildings such as the Paint and Trunnel Shop (where paints and finishes used on wooden ships were manufactured), the Mill and Joiner Shop (where cabin interiors were produced), and the Oakum Shop (where the caulkers stored their materials). The Small Craft Center houses an extensive collection of classic boats, along with the apprenticeshop.

At "Lobstering and the Maine Coast," a major exhibit detailing the story of lobster history and technology from colonial times to the present, you'll learn that lobsters were once so plentiful that colonists could simply reach out and catch them with a gaff in the shallow water. Whereas five-footers were

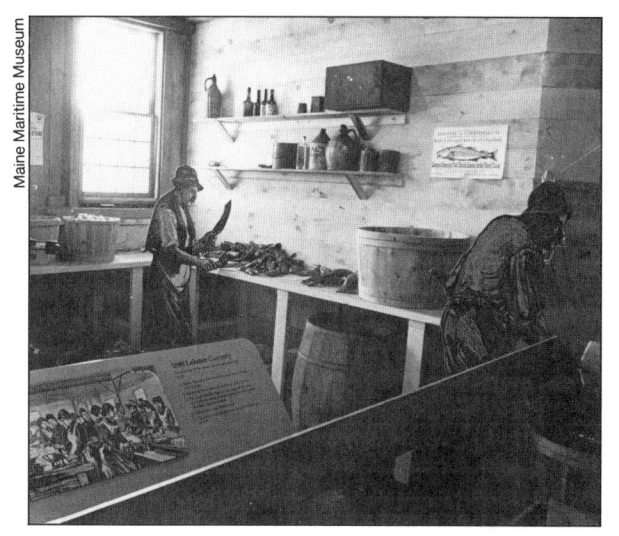

The lobsterman in this historical exhibit at the Maine Maritime Museum "talks" to you about his life and work and about the rewards of being his own boss.

common in those days, even one-footers are rare now. The exhibit includes a mockup of an 1880s vintage lobster cannery. Back then, as now, Maine was plagued with seasonal unemployment problems. A century ago the Maine canneries employed about 782 people, 349 of them women and children. The men earned $6 to $15 per week, and the women and children got $3 to $4. But the canning season lasted only four months, which meant a woman could make only about $70 a year. A 1979 study showed that the average lobsterman still put out a lot of effort for a limited return, netting only $800 a month.

The exhibit includes a diorama where a mannequin of a lobsterman talks about his life. He explains the work involved in trapping lobsters — getting up at 5 A.M., using 600 traps to capture as many lobsters as he used to be able to get with 150. He talks too about the rewards of being his own boss.

You can sit in a lobster boat and watch an eighteen-minute video describing the life of the lobsterman, whose office is a boat and whose calendar shows his engagements with the tides. You can also examine a collection of lobster boats, bait barrels, trap hawlers, toggles, buoys, traps, and related equipment.

While at the shipyard, climb aboard the Grand Banks schooner *Sherman Zwicker*. Approximately 400,000 pounds of cod were cleaned and salted down for trips home aboard the schooner's deck during its forays into the North Atlantic from 1942 to 1968. Visit the engine house, the crew's quarters, and the dory fishing exhibit in the hold. Take a look at the original logbook. According to Captain Pitwood

Lobsters were once so plentiful that colonists could simply reach out and catch them with a gaff in the shallow water.

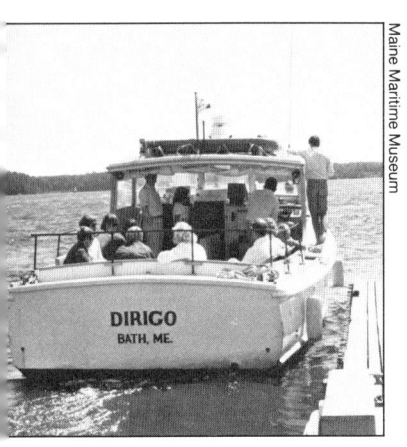

When you've finished with the exhibits at the shipyard, take a forty-minute ride along the Kennebec River aboard the Dirigo.

Maine Maritime Museum

Park's notations, 450 lines were fished and 40,000 pounds of cod harvested on November 11, 1955.

When you've finished with the exhibits at the shipyard, take a forty-minute ride along the Kennebec aboard the *Dirigo*. The cruise provides an excellent vantage point for viewing the waterfront, including activity at Bath Iron Works. That 400-foot-high crane you see can pick up loads weighing 220 tons, swinging them a full 360 degrees. The trip originates and ends at the shipyard.

A free shuttle bus will take you to the museum's in-town site, the **Sewall House**. This 1844 mansion was once the home of one of Bath's foremost shipbuilding families. Here you'll see extensive collections of marine art, half models, navigational instruments, and sailors' mementos. Other exhibits provide insight into the lives of shipbuilding and seafaring families, while still others focus on the history of Bath Iron Works. There are detailed dioramas, too, including one of the Sewall Shipyard with its tiny vessels in various stages of construction.

Allow several hours to experience the Maine Maritime Museum, perhaps beginning your day or breaking up your visit with a leisurely meal at **Kristina's,** a cheerful restaurant that can satisfy just about any taste at almost any time of day. Eat outside on the porch in fair weather, or settle down indoors in a wooden booth in the informal blue-and-white room, where you can have breakfast or lunch. For dinner, pass through the lace-curtained doors into the dining room, where a vase of fresh flowers decorates each table. Live entertainment is sometimes featured in the second-story lounge.

Breakfast is always noteworthy at Kristina's, but Sunday brunch is fabulous. Every dish has a special touch. The French toast is made with cinnamon swirl bread, and the three types of pancakes (honey bran, buttermilk, and plain) are served with your choice of blueberries, sautéed cinnamon and apples, or sliced bananas. Also available are omelettes, quiches, and special dishes such as Seafood Benedict (poached eggs on a grilled English muffin with sautéed scallions, shrimp, and haddock broiled with Swiss cheese and hollandaise). Treat yourself to a steaming cup of espresso, cappuccino, or mochaccino — available in decaffeinated, too.

For lunch and dinner you can choose a light meal such as a charbroiled burger, Spanakopita (spinach and feta cheese filling baked in a flaky phyllo crust), and Tourtière (French Canadian pork pie baked in a Cheddar cheese crust). The inventive entrées vary from Tenderloin in Bordelaise with Mushroom Caps to Honey Mustard Chicken, from Shrimp and Scallop Marinara to Vegetable Alfredo (spinach pasta with fresh vegetables in a sauce of heavy cream, fresh garlic, and Parmesan cheese). Wines and beers are available. Kristina's also has its own bakery, and you ought to take a look in the pastry case before making a dessert choice.

If you would prefer to put together a picnic, perhaps to eat at one of the benches along the Kennebec down at Waterfront Park on Commercial Street, try **The Granary,** a natural foods store that puts up containers of homemade soups such as lentil, minestrone, and carrot cashew. Add a couple of homemade muffins or a Havacado sandwich (Havarti cheese and avocado) and you've got a healthy, inexpensive lunch to take out or eat at one of the small tables on the raised platforms by The Granary's windows.

After lunch take a walk along Front Street. Bath's main thoroughfare has been restored nineteenth-century style, with period light fixtures, brick sidewalks, and bright awnings. You might run across Mr. Popcorn, with his old-fashioned yellow-and-red cart with the glass box full of freshly popped kernels. He even offers a senior citizen discount. On Saturdays from June through October, the atmosphere resembles a street fair, the sidewalks lined with craft tables and food booths. Craft demonstrations and street entertainment often are part of the fun.

Speaking of crafts, stop in at Front Street's **Yankee Artisan,** where glazed honey pots, fluted pie plates, mugs, candlesticks, and vases by New England craftspeople perch on crates and open shelves. Rainbow-colored rag rugs hang on wooden wall racks, and small braided rugs are piled high in an old crib. There are warm woolen hand-knit socks and sweaters and delicate hand-smocked christening dresses, clipboards decorated with pigs, patchwork aprons, stenciled totes, and goat's milk fudge packaged in pretty baskets.

Serious home handymen might be interested in visiting **Shelter Institute,** famous for its rigorous course that teaches people to design, build, or retrofit an energy-efficient home. If you are interested in the course, ask to see the slide show that details the hands-on shelter instructional approach. This is also the place to search out those hard-to-find tools necessary for fine woodworking projects. At **Woodbutcher Tools,** a division of the institute located in

Bath's main thoroughfare has been restored nineteenth-century style, with period light fixtures, brick sidewalks, and bright awnings.

The founding of Bath Iron Works in 1894 enabled the city to keep abreast of changes in shipbuilding technology. Here a ship is launched from the iron works.

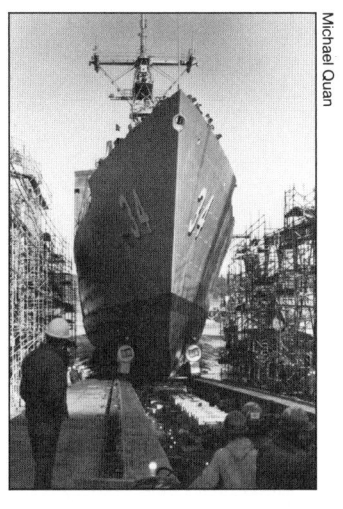

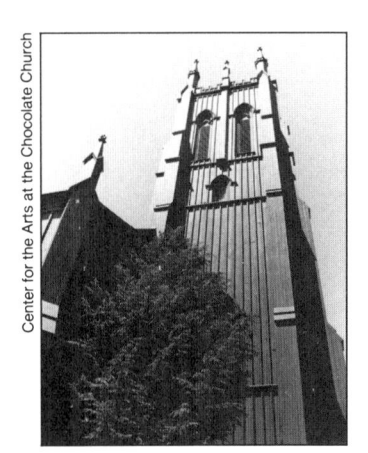

The Chocolate Church, a Bath landmark, features an art gallery and a theater.

the same building, you'll see Marples chisels, Murphy shop knives, Smiths pocket stones, and hundreds of other tools and accessories.

Another important Bath landmark is the **Center for the Arts at the Chocolate Church,** which has its own art gallery as well as a theater for plays and dance performances. The old church frequently echoes with music, ranging from classical to bluegrass to folk. Write or call ahead for a schedule to help you plan your visit.

ACCESS

BATH. Follow I-95 to Portland, then take Route 1 north to the Bath Business District exit.

MAINE MARITIME MUSEUM. Directions: Take the Bath Business District exit from Route 1. Turn south at lights and follow signs 1¼ miles to free parking at museum shipyard. **Season:** Year-round; shipyard closes mid-October. Shuttle bus operates between shipyard and Sewall House from late June through early September. **Admission:** Charged; senior discount. **Telephone:** (207) 443-1316.

KRISTINA'S. Directions: Located at 160 Center Street. **Season:** Year-round. **Admission:** Free. **Telephone:** (207) 442-8577.

THE GRANARY. Directions: Located on Center Street, adjacent to Shelter Institute. **Season:** Year-round. **Admission:** Free. **Telephone:** (207) 442-8012.

YANKEE ARTISAN. Directions: Located at 178 Front Street. **Season:** Year-round. **Admission:** Free. **Telephone:** (207) 443-6215.

SHELTER INSTITUTE. Directions: Located at 38 Center Street. **Season:** Year-round. **Admission:** Free. **Telephone:** (207) 442-7938.

CENTER FOR THE ARTS AT THE CHOCOLATE CHURCH. Directions: Located at 804 Washington Street. **Season:** Year-round. **Admission:** Charged. **Telephone:** (207) 442-8455.

For further information or restaurant and lodging suggestions, contact the Bath Area Chamber of Commerce, 45 Front Street, Bath, ME 04530. Telephone: (207) 443-9751.

Castine

A classic New England seaside village, Castine cleaves to the tip of a finger of land extending out into Penobscot Bay. You'll travel past saltwater farms and simple houses, broad meadows and stretches of the Penobscot River as you drive the fifteen miles leading from the main road to the town. Along the way you might see a sign saying "Please drive slowly — geese at play," or another advertising the availability of homemade preserves.

Castine is endowed with a lovely harbor, a lively history, and a main street that looks like it slipped off a postcard. Settle in at a local inn for a weekend or a week or enroll in an Elderhostel program. Sample fresh seafood, shop for local crafts, improve your golf swing, or go to the theater, all without leaving town.

Castine, unlike many resort towns, is seldom overrun with visitors. It offers plenty to see and do, but there are no crowds. There is also no particular spot to get information, but that's not really a problem. Posters announcing events and activities are taped to store windows, providing you with up-to-date information on everything from barn sales to guided nature walks.

As you enter town, you'll drive through the middle of the nine-hole golf course belonging to the **Castine Golf Club.** The course dates back to 1897 and is open to the public. The clubhouse is within easy walking distance of the village green, the waterfront, and the shopping area. Check in for a couple of days at a local inn and play golf without ever having to climb into your car — just about as convenient as you can get.

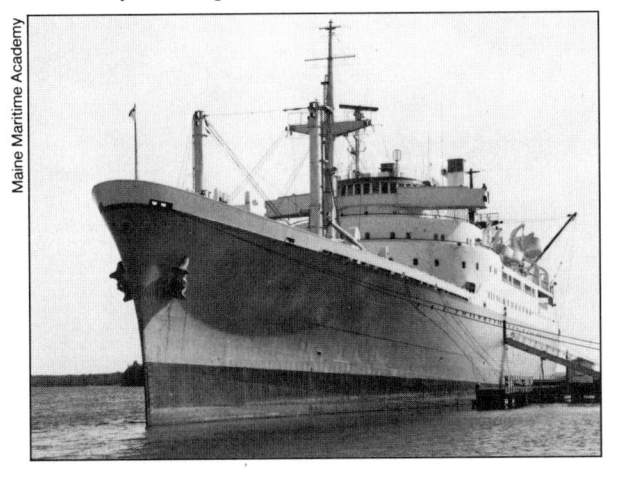

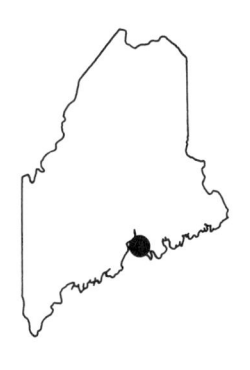

Tours of the 7,000-ton training vessel, State of Maine, *are conducted whenever the ship is in port, which is most of the time.*

Named for the Frenchman Baron de Castin, the village of Castine has been under the rule of four different nations — Britain, France, Holland, and the United States.

After crossing the golf course, bear left and continue down Main Street to the wharves (complete with public rest rooms). Your eyes will be drawn to the huge *State of Maine,* the seven-thousand-ton ship used as a training vessel for students at the Maine Maritime Academy. It dwarfs all the other boats in sight. Visitors are taken on tours of the ship whenever it is in port, which is most of the time. Be prepared for lots of walking and stairs.

To get right out on the water, take a one-and-a-half-hour cruise with **Castine Harbor Tours** along the shores of Penobscot Bay. Your tour will take you past revolutionary war sites of importance such as Trask Rock and Blockhouse Point, and your captain will explain their significance. You'll also cruise along the edge of the **Holbrook Wildlife Sanctuary,** where harbor seals and osprey often come to feed. Since the boat accommodates only six passengers at a time, you'll feel more like a guest than a paying customer.

Plan to have at least one meal down on the wharves watching the elegant sailboats slide by. **The Breeze,** a take-out stand, offers fresh crab rolls, clam and haddock dinners, burgers, and sandwiches. There's a wooden deck with picnic tables perched right over the harbor where you can settle comfortably with your purchase.

For a fancier meal, try **Dennett's Wharf,** a complex that includes a spacious, pleasant dining room offering full-course dinners, cocktails, and a raw bar. Dine indoors or out on the open deck, where blue-and-white Cinzano umbrellas make each table look like a huge flower in bloom. There's a market selling fine wines and beers, fresh lobster meat, fish, fruit, cold cuts, and bread. This is a good place to assemble a picnic lunch. If you're heading home from Castine, you can get live lobsters "packed to travel"; they'll be fine for twenty-four hours. Dennett's Wharf also offers dockage to visiting mariners, and it's fun to watch new arrivals tie up below.

Speaking of picnics, **Castine Creations** will prepare a lovely one for you. A sample dinner includes shrimp cocktail, fresh-picked mussels, lobster salad, cucumber sandwiches, dessert, and a beverage. You'll have to call a day and a half ahead to order your picnic. Although seafood is a specialty, chicken dishes are available as well. Castine Creations makes two soups of the day, one hot and one cold, from carrot bisque to shrimp gumbo. Order by the pint or quart, as an addition to your picnic or as a light meal of its own.

As you gaze out over the boats bobbing in the bay, bear in mind that there was a time when you needed a boat just to get to Castine. That was back when the British were in control of the village. In 1779, as part of their defense system, they hand-dug a canal, severing Castine from the mainland. This is but one incident in the town's colorful history.

Named for the Frenchman Baron de Castin, who used the site as his headquarters and trading post in the mid-seventeenth century, the village of Castine has been under the rule of four different nations — Britain, France, Holland, and the United States. It changed hands among the four no fewer than nine times, a record unequaled by any other settlement in Maine. In the course of its history, Castine suffered frequent burnings and pillagings, so although it has been around since 1629 when the Plymouth Pilgrims first established it as a trading post named Bagaduce, there are fewer old buildings and historic landmarks than you might expect. Yet the town is peppered with historical plaques, more than a hundred of them, describing important and intriguing moments in Castine's history.

For example, **Petty's Pizza,** an unassuming, small, gray-shingled building, has a plaque that reads: "On May 8, 1768, this was declared the first condemned building in North America." Today it's a good place to have a hearty and economical breakfast, lunch, or dinner. Of course there's pizza (made on a white or whole wheat crust), but that's just the beginning. Take a seat at the small counter or in one of the booths and get serious about breakfast. Have an omelette, a stack of blueberry pancakes, a slab of Canadian bacon, or maybe a serving of baked beans. Later in the day feast on a down-home meal like meat loaf or chicken Parmesan with spaghetti. Or opt for chowder or calzone. As for drinks, you can choose from twenty kinds of beer.

Getting back to history, you can wander through the ruins of **Fort George,** the last British holding to be surrendered to American forces at the end of the American Revolution. During the War of 1812, it was briefly revived as a British outpost. The ruins of the old fort sit behind the Maine Maritime Academy, which was built on the site of the old British barracks.

A rainy afternoon can be well spent pursuing local history via visits to the **John Perkins House,** of particular appeal to those interested in eighteenth-century architecture, and the **Wilson Museum**. At the latter you'll see exhibits of artifacts relating to the

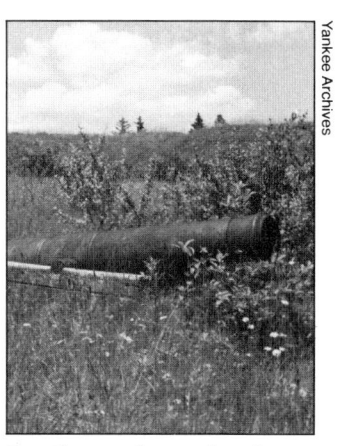

Fort George, the remains of which sit behind the Maine Maritime Academy, was the last British holding surrendered to American forces at the end of the American Revolution.

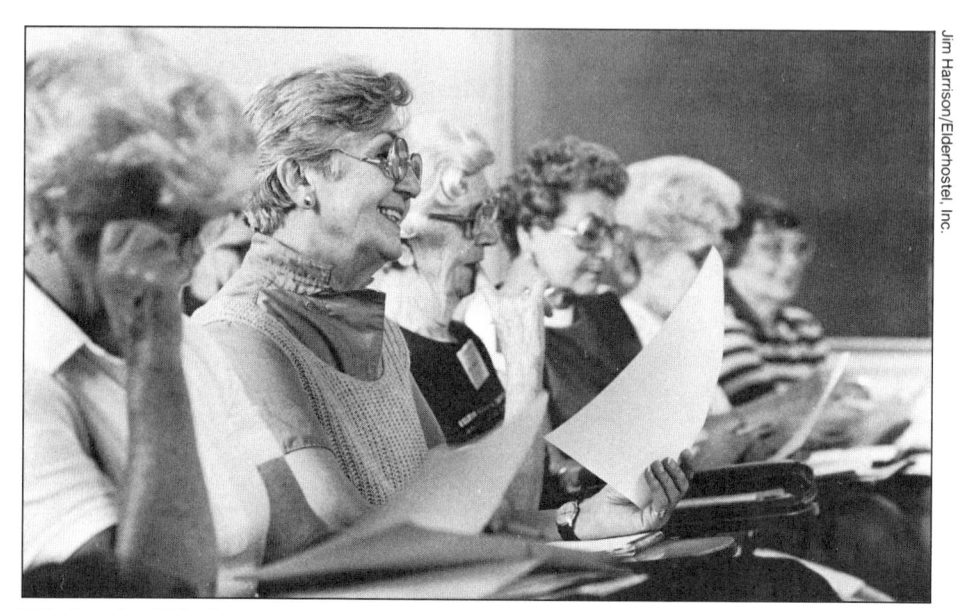

Elderhostel, which offers courses throughout New England, operates a program at Castine's Maine Maritime Academy.

Paleolithic, Neolithic, Bronze, and Iron ages. In keeping with the town's turbulent military history, the museum also houses a collection of early guns and firearms.

For a quick trip back into Castine's past, you need only take a walk around the lovely village green, shaded by huge old trees and early American buildings. The **Old Meeting House,** built in 1790, has a Bulfinch steeple and a bell cast by Paul Revere. It is one of the oldest churches in Maine. Most years the local merchants get together and publish a free walking tour map, describing the historic buildings. If you would like to have one, stop in at one of the stores and inquire.

Main Street, which runs down to the waterfront, and Water Street, which crosses it and runs parallel to the wharves, are lined with interesting shops. **Simple Pleasures of Maine** sells Maine-made items, consigned by fifty craftspeople, including quilts, sweaters, stenciled linen table mats, wooden toys, puzzles, and even handmade game knives. The shop also sells art and needlework supplies. Linda and Susan, the enthusiastic proprietors, sponsor frequent miniworkshops on subjects such as printing, knitting, and several styles of rug making. This is a pleasant, unpressured place to learn a new skill or refresh an old one.

You may also want to enroll in an **Elderhostel** program based at the Maine Maritime Academy. As with all Elderhostel programs, the fee covers accommodations (in Maritime Academy housing), all meals, and tuition costs. Courses change from year to year but are likely to include Archaeology of Penobscot Bay Focusing on Castine, which concentrates on changes that have taken place in the native culture over the past twelve thousand years by examining the rich archaeological evidence found in Maine. If you have always wanted to learn to sail but have never gotten around to it, enroll in Basic Sailing and Navigation, which covers all aspects of small-boat handling, combining lectures with hands-on experience. The course, which is designed for inexperienced sailors, uses sixteen-foot Mercury-class sailboats.

If you would like to familiarize yourself with local flora and fauna, join one of the guided nature walks frequently offered in the summer months by the **Castine Conservation Trust**. You might go looking for lichens behind Fort George or searching for wildflowers on the back shore. Birding at Hatch Cove's sandbar is another possibility. Call ahead for information or check the posters in the stores.

If you would like to take a swim, head for the small beach located about half a mile from the Maritime Academy. There are no commercial establishments in sight, just a couple of white houses and, across the bay, a red barn. Park your car by the road just steps from the rocky stretch of beach. The water is quiet, and there is marshy land across the road, making this an altogether peaceful spot.

In the evening you can attend a play by the **Cold Comfort Productions** summer theater. Performances are conveniently held right in the village, at the Maine Maritime Academy auditorium. A recent season saw productions of *Side by Side, Oliver, The Six Wives of Henry the VIII,* and a serious contemporary work called *Extremities*.

For a quick trip into Castine's past, you need only take a walk around the lovely village green, shaded by huge old trees and early American buildings.

ACCESS

CASTINE. Follow Route 1 to Orland. Take Route 175 south to Route 166, then follow Route 166 into the center of town. It is 15 miles from Orland to Castine.

CASTINE GOLF CLUB. Directions: Located on Battle Avenue (Route 166) in Castine. **Season:** Late spring through fall. **Admission:** Greens fee charged. **Telephone:** (207) 326-8844.

STATE OF MAINE. **Directions:** Docked in Castine Harbor, adjacent to the town wharf. **Season:** Year-round, except May and June. **Admission:** Free. **Telephone:** (207) 326-4311.

CASTINE HARBOR TOURS. Directions: Turn left on Main Street off Route 166 and continue to bottom of street, where Main and Water Streets intersect. Located at 1 Water Street in Castine. **Season:** June through September. **Admission:** Charged. **Telephone:** (207) 326-9494. **Note:** Tours by reservation only.

THE BREEZE. Directions: Located on the town wharf. Wharf is located just beyond the intersection of Main and Water streets. **Season:** Memorial Day through Labor Day. **Admission:** Free. **Telephone:** None.

DENNETT'S WHARF. Directions: Located on the waterfront in Castine. **Season:** Memorial Day through mid-September. **Admission:** Free. **Telephone:** (207) 326-9045.

CASTINE CREATIONS. Directions: Call to order picnics. **Season:** Memorial Day through Labor Day. **Telephone:** (207) 326-8664.

PETTY'S PIZZA. Directions: Located on Water Street. **Season:** Year-round. **Admission:** Free. **Telephone:** (207) 326-4047.

FORT GEORGE. Directions: Located across from the Maine Maritime Academy on Route 166, just beyond the golf club. **Season:** Year-round. **Admission:** Free. **Telephone:** None.

JOHN PERKINS HOUSE. Directions: Located next to Wilson Museum. **Season:** July and August. **Admission:** Free. **Telephone:** None.

WILSON MUSEUM. Directions: Traveling into town on Route 166, turn left on Main Street (faces the golf club). Take the second right, onto Perkins Street, where the museum is located. **Season:** July and August. **Admission:** Free. **Telephone:** None.

SIMPLE PLEASURES OF MAINE. Directions: Located at 1 Water Street in Castine. **Season:** Year-round. **Admission:** Free. **Telephone:** (207) 326-8861.

ELDERHOSTEL. Directions: Program is located at the Maine Maritime Academy in the center of Castine. **Season:** Late July through early August. **Admission:** Charged. **Telephone:** (617) 426-8056. **Note:** For a complete catalog of courses, write Elderhostel, 80 Boylston Street, Suite 400, Boston, MA 02116.

CASTINE CONSERVATION TRUST. Directions: Trips assemble in front of the town hall on Court Street in Castine. **Season:** Late June through August. **Admission:** Free. **Telephone:** None. **Note:** For a schedule, write to the Castine Conservation Trust, Box 421, Castine, ME 04421.

COLD COMFORT PRODUCTIONS. Directions: Performances held in Maine Maritime Academy auditorium. **Season:** Mid-July through August. **Admission:** Charged. **Telephone:** (207) 326-9041.

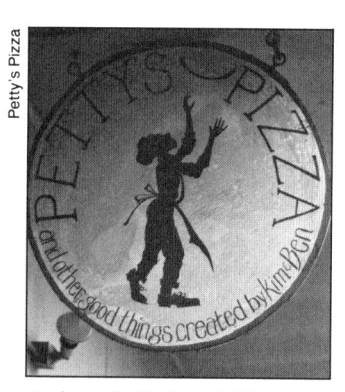

A plaque in the Petty's Pizza building reads: "On May 8, 1768, this was declared the first condemned building in North America." Things have been all uphill since.

Blue Hill

Blue Hill, situated halfway down the Penobscot Peninsula, is a prosperous coastal community with an artistic bent. Stonington, located about twenty-five miles south of Blue Hill at the southern tip of Deer Isle, is an archetypal Maine fishing village, with Jericho Bay and a cluster of tiny islands as a backdrop. The stretch of road between the two is perfect territory for those who enjoy the classic "Sunday drive."

Stonington, reached by a bridge across Eggemoggin Reach, is forty miles away from well-trafficked coastal Route 1. Yet those forty miles feel more like four hundred. Actually, miles don't mean much here. You can't go very fast, and you won't want to anyhow. There's too much to enjoy in this maze of peninsulas and islands, an exquisite, unspoiled appendage of coastal Maine.

Perhaps it is the drama of the natural environment that makes this part of Maine a mecca for those who take joy in creating something beautiful with their hands and hearts, be it music, art, craft, or garden. Whether you're looking to join in the creating or just to admire the creations of others, this region will satisfy you.

Blue Hill has long been associated with fine music because of the **Kneisel Hall** chamber music school. The school presents concerts throughout the summer and also sponsors special events, such as the recent "Evening of Airs, Madrigals and Other Vocal Delights."

Blue Hill and the tiny villages on Deer Isle are also home to many attractive galleries. Artist Judith Leighton shows her own work at Blue Hill's **Leighton Gallery,** one of Maine's most successful galleries. Her paintings are gentle, intimate, and colorful, traits she also tends to favor in the work of other artists she exhibits. **The Handworks Gallery,** also in Blue Hill, specializes in fine contemporary crafts, including furniture, pottery, handwoven clothing, baskets, rugs, jewelry, and blown glass. At neighboring **Cole House Quilts,** Amish and Mennonite quilts are displayed in bedroom settings. Here too you'll find quilts that reflect fresh interpretations of traditional designs. Works by many local artists are featured at the **Turtle Gallery**, perched right on the edge of the harbor in tiny Deer Isle Village. As its name indicates, the **Eastern Bay Cooperative Gallery** on the waterfront in Stonington is a joint venture, owned and operated by the fifty Maine artisans and artists

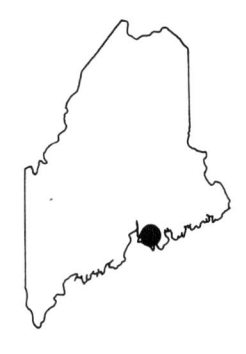

You can't go very fast, and you won't want to anyhow. There's too much to enjoy.

who exhibit here. Handmade pieces cover the spectrum from purely decorative to utilitarian, reflecting a broad range of media, workmanship, and styles.

These shops and galleries are only a start; there are lots of others, and you are sure to find your own favorites.

To see artisans at work, be sure to visit **Rowantrees Pottery**. As founder Adelaide Pearson used to say, "Just come up the garden path and visit the pottery." Named for the mountain ash trees that shade its gate, Rowantrees Pottery got its start in 1934. Even today, every piece is handmade on the potter's wheel, and all you need to do is follow the brick path to the studio door. The potters are always willing to demonstrate their skill, so if they are not working when you arrive, just speak up and tell them that you'd like to see a pot thrown.

Working with native clay, the two resident potters deftly form and define the graceful pieces of earthenware. Depending on when you drop in, you might find bare pieces of fired pottery and trays of partially finished jam jar tops or craftspeople skillfully applying glazes to the pitchers, plates, mugs, and bowls that have already had their first baking in the hot kilns.

Rowantrees pottery is glazed in turquoise, oyster white, evergreen, jonquil yellow, moss agate, duckshead, and heather blue, as you'll see when you climb the stairs to the large second-story showroom. There are also two-tone pieces done in duckshead with turquoise, duckshead with moss agate, heather blue with white, and black with sea gull. Because the colors complement each other, you can mix and match endlessly to satisfy your own tastes.

The product line itself offers numerous possibilities, too. Plates come in five sizes, as do cups and saucers. The line of serving pieces and accessories runs the gamut from soufflé dishes to soup tureens, butter dishes to bean pots, along with candleholders, trivets, wine coolers, bells, and bud vases. The most popular item is the jam jar set, crowned with a spray of hand-formed blueberries or strawberries.

Professional artisan, serious amateur, and neophyte share their affection and respect for craft media each summer at the **Haystack Mountain School of Crafts** on Deer Isle. During the two- and three-week residential sessions, students live, study, and work together in a self-contained community overlooking sparkling Jericho Bay, sprinkled with lobster boats and tiny pine-studded islands. The "community" is, in fact, a series of wooden decks, on which are

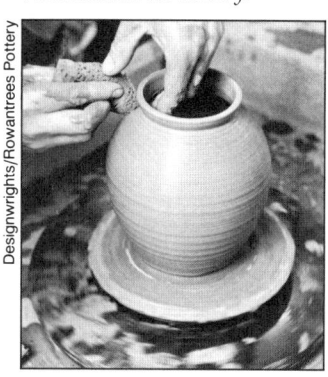

To see artisans at work, be sure to visit Rowantrees Pottery.

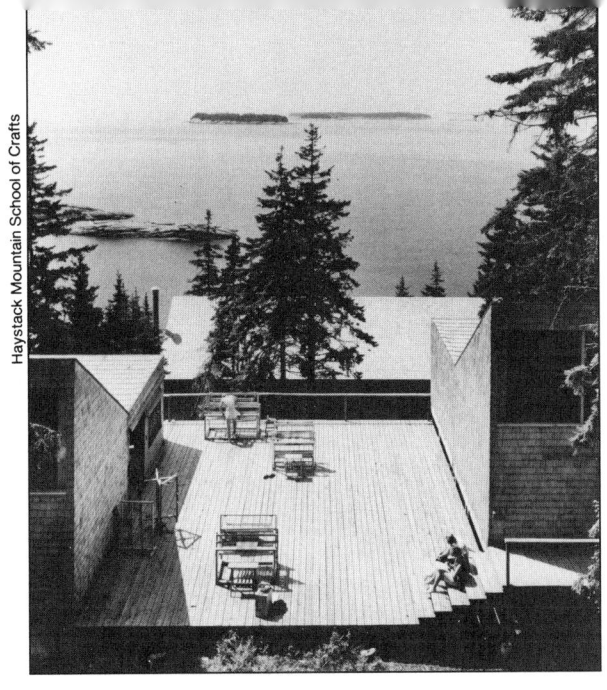

With sparkling Jericho Bay as its backdrop, Deer Isle's Haystack Mountain School of Crafts provides a one-of-a-kind learning experience.

built shingled studios and cabins. The songs of birds, the hum of boat engines, and the lap of the ocean mingle with voices and the sounds of tools at work.

At Haystack, you'll live in a comfortable double or triple cabin. Participants share communal meals in the dining room, and evenings are enriched by a variety of programs presented by visiting artists and performers. The outdoor six-sided wooden stage is canopied by evergreens, and the area around the rows of log benches is carpeted with moss and pine needles.

To put it simply, Haystack offers an intense experience. Studios are open around the clock, every day of the week, with classes scheduled Monday through Friday. Applicants are chosen on the basis of a short statement of intent, describing their background and what they hope to accomplish during the session. Applicants for courses requiring previous experience must submit slides of their work. Each participant chooses one medium or "studio" for the whole session. Studios are offered in baskets, blacksmithing, clay, metals, sequential imagery, surface design, fibers, glass blowing, quilts, wood, drawing and painting, woodturning, and paper.

Anyone eighteen or older can apply to Haystack, which means there is a great diversity in the ages, backgrounds, and experiences that participants bring to Deer Isle. If you enjoy mingling with younger people as well as those your own age, and if the idea of several weeks of intense concentration on a craft in a magnificent rural island setting sounds

Professional artisan, serious amateur, and neophyte share their affection and respect for craft media each summer at the Haystack Mountain School of Crafts on Deer Isle.

like your idea of heaven, write for a complete catalog. Although students are accepted right up until the day a course begins, applications are processed in the order in which they are received, so it's best to apply by April 15 if you have your heart set on a specific studio.

Visitors are welcome at Haystack. If you do not wish to apply for admission to a studio but would like to get a closer look, plan to visit between 10 A.M. and 4 P.M., Thursday through Sunday. Visitors may also attend the evening programs, usually scheduled for 8:30 P.M., and the auctions of student work held at the close of each session. Call the school for dates and details.

For a close look at a very different form of creative expression, visit **Meadow House.** Roseanne and Joe Dombek have been gardening right here in Blue Hill since 1971. Their interest in herbs was originally generated by a priest who showed them how to use the plants in French cooking. They've been growing herbs ever since, and they currently cultivate about three hundred varieties.

What sets Meadow House apart from other herb businesses is that you can wander through the gardens. Not only will you go home with sweet-smelling plants, but you'll find yourself laden with practical ideas you can apply to your own garden plans. Unlike formal gardens maintained by a professional staff, the Dombeks' gardens are the kind you can duplicate with your own efforts.

There are twelve separate gardens, each with a different theme. If you want to re-create one of the designs at home, you can purchase a diagram so you know just what plants are called for and where to put them. If you like to make your own potpourri or dried flower arrangements, take a good look at the cut flower garden and the everlasting garden. Cooks will be intrigued by both by the culinary garden and the libation garden, the latter chock-full of elderberry bushes, hops, grapevines, sweet woodruff, and mint. Some others are the gray-green garden, the spring bulb garden, and the fragrant garden. Throughout the plantings you'll find gazebos and trellises, birdbaths and benches, along with whimsical bits of statuary like the curly-haired fellow munching handfuls of grapes in the libation garden.

The walls in the cozy Herb Shop are covered with bouquets of dried flowers and delicate wreaths fashioned from herbs. Coils of bittersweet and grapevines hang from the rafters. The culinary corner includes dozens of herbs for cooking, along with

The walls in the cozy herb shop are covered with bouquets of dried flowers and delicate wreaths fashioned from herbs.

teapots and other gifts. One of Roseanne's handmade herb hot mats makes a nice remembrance. She stuffs each pretty calico mat with culinary herbs such as cinnamon, marjoram, and oregano. When you put a hot pot of tea on the mat, the heat releases the heady scent of the herbs beneath. There's also a small Plant Shop, which sells gardening supplies. Do-it-yourselfers will find Meadow House a good source of handy supplies and generous advice, whether you want to grow herbs, make your own potpourri and wreaths, or do it all.

ACCESS

BLUE HILL. Follow Route 1 north to Bucksport. Turn right on Route 15 and continue into Blue Hill.

DEER ISLE. Follow Route 15 south from Blue Hill, crossing a bridge and a causeway.

KNEISEL HALL. Directions: Located on Pleasant Street (Route 15) in Blue Hill. **Season:** Late June through August. **Admission:** Charged. **Telephone:** (207) 374-2811.

LEIGHTON GALLERY. Directions: Located on Parker Point Road in Blue Hill. Follow Route 15 to Main Street, where it joins Route 176. Turn right on Main Street (Routes 176/15), then left on Parker Point Road. **Season:** May through mid-October; Thanksgiving through Christmas. **Admission:** Free. **Telephone:** (207) 374-5001.

THE HANDWORKS GALLERY. Directions: Located on Main Street (Routes 176/15) in Blue Hill. **Season:** May through October. **Admission:** Free. **Telephone:** (207) 374-5613.

COLE HOUSE QUILTS. Directions: Located on Union Street (Route 177) in Blue Hill. **Season:** May through Christmas; closed one week in mid-October. **Admission:** Free. **Telephone:** (207) 374-2175.

TURTLE GALLERY. Directions: Located at 219 Deer Isle Village, which straddles Route 15, on Deer Isle. **Season:**

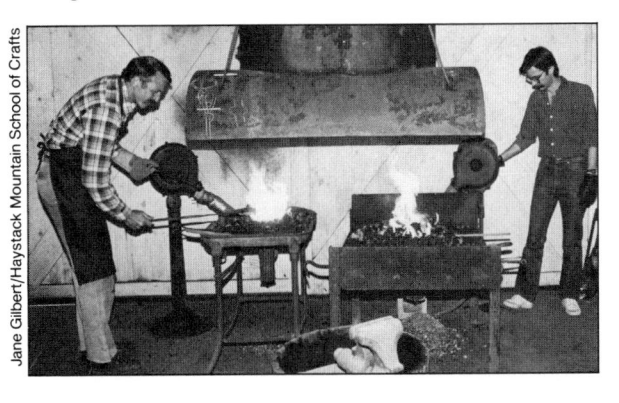

Forging ahead! The Haystack Mountain School of Crafts offers an "intense" experience with studios open around the clock.

May through October. **Admission:** Free. **Telephone:** (207) 348-9977.

EASTERN BAY COOPERATIVE GALLERY. Directions: From Blue Hill, follow Route 15 south to Stonington. Located on Main Street. **Season:** May through October; Thanksgiving through Christmas. **Admission:** Free. **Telephone:** (207) 367-5006.

ROWANTREES POTTERY. Directions: Entering Blue Hill traveling south on Route 15, turn right on Union Street (Route 177). Rowantrees is located on the left at 9 Union Street. **Season:** Year-round. **Admission:** Free. **Telephone:** (207) 374-5535.

HAYSTACK MOUNTAIN SCHOOL OF CRAFTS. Directions: Follow Route 15 south, crossing the bridge to Deer Isle. Continue about 5 miles on Route 15, past Deer Isle Village. Turn left at the Gulf station and follow the small white "Haystack" signs for about 7 miles to the school. **Season:** June through September; open to visitors Thursday through Sunday. **Admission:** Free; program fees. **Telephone:** (207) 348-2306.

MEADOW HOUSE. Directions: Entering Blue Hill traveling south on Route 15, turn right on Union Street (Route 177), following signs to Meadow House. **Season:** April through December. **Admission:** Free. **Telephone:** (207) 374-5043.

For further information or restaurant and lodging suggestions, contact the Blue Hill Chamber of Commerce, P.O. Box 520, Blue Hill, ME 04614.

Index

Alley Beat, The, 133, 136
All Language Programs. *See* ALPS
ALPS, 109, 111
American Precision Museum, 120-121, 123-124
Andrews Point, 67, 70
Annalee's Gift Shop and Museum, 90-91, 93
Antiques, 25, 91-92, 113-114, 116. *See also* Auctions; Historic sites; Museums
Auctions, 71-72
Audubon Society, 18-19, 20, 21, 153, 155

Back Beach, 67
Baker Library, 108-109, 111
Bartholomew's Cobble, 73-74, 75
Bascom Lodge, 81, 83
Basin, The, 96
Bath, Maine, 156-160
Battery Park, 147, 149
Beantown Trolleys, 51, 54
Belle of Brattleboro, 113, 118
Ben & Jerry's, 147, 149
Birdcraft Museum and Sanctuary, 19, 21
Blue Hill, Maine, 167-172
Boise Rock, 96-97
Boston, Massachusetts, 47-54
Boston Harbor Cruises, 54
Boston Tea Party Ship and Museum, The, 50, 54
Bowen House, 21-24, 27
Bradford Galleries, Ltd., 71-72, 75
Brattleboro, Vermont, 112-119
Breeze, The, 162, 166
Brookfield, Connecticut, 28-33
Brookfield Craft Center, 28-30, 33
Brush Hill Tours, 49-51, 53-54
Buell's Greenhouses, 24-25, 27
Bunker Hill Pavilion, 51, 54
Burlington, Vermont, 144-149
Burr Mansion, 18

Calvin Coolidge Homestead, 129, 130
Cannon Mountain Ski Area, 97-98, 99
Cannon Tram II, 97, 98, 99
Canterbury, New Hampshire, 84-87

Captain Ted's Rockport Whale Watching, 68, 70
Carousel Candies, 46, 47
Castine, Maine, 161-166
Castine Conservation Trust, 165, 166
Castine Creations, 162, 166
Castine Golf Club, 161, 165
Castine Harbor Tours, 162, 166
Center for the Arts at the Chocolate Church, 160
Champlain Chocolate, 144-145, 148
Champlain Shakespeare Festival, 141, 146, 148-149
Charlotte, Vermont, 143
Charlotte-Essex Ferry, 142, 143
Cheese Outlet, 145-146, 148
Chocolate Church, Center for the Arts at the, 160
Christmas in Rockport, 69, 70
Christmas Pageant, Annual, 69
Church Street Marketplace, 147, 149
Clark Art Institute, Sterling and Francine, 76-77, 82
Classes, 30-31, 41, 109, 159, 164-165. *See Also* Workshops
Coach Barn, 139-140
Cold Comfort Productions, 165, 166
Cole House Quilts, 167, 171
College Bookstore, The, 78, 79, 82-83
Colonel Ashley House, 74-75, 76
Colonial Craft Day, 16-17
Connecticut, 15-33
Connecticut Audubon Society Fairfield Center, 18-19, 20
Constitution, USS, 49, 50-51, 53, 54
Constitution House, 120, 123
Constitution Museum, USS, 49, 51, 53, 54
Corn Crib, The, 73, 75
Crafts, 16-17, 28-30, 72, 87, 109-110, 121-122, 126, 128-129, 132-133, 154-155, 159, 164, 167-170. *See also* Shopping
Craftsbury Chamber Players, 146-147, 149
Crowninshield-Bentley House, 57-58

Dartmouth College Hopkins Center, 107, 111
Daytrips. *See* Trips-at-a-Glance
Decoy Shop, The, 154-155, 155-156
Deer Isle, Maine, 167-172
Dennett's Wharf, 162, 166
Dogwood Festival, Annual, 17
Downstairs at the Playhouse, 126, 130
Dutton Berry Farm, 114, 118

Dutton Farm Stand, 114, 118
Eastern Bay Cooperative Gallery, 167-168, 172
East Matunuck State Beach, 38, 39
Echo Lake, 84, 99
Elderhostel, 9-10, 164-165, 166
Erasmus Café, 78-79, 82-83
Essex Institute, 57-58, 62
Extended Stays, 12, 28-33, 40-70, 76-83, 94-119, 124-143, 150-156, 161-172

Fairfield, Connecticut, 15-21
Fairfield Historical Society, 15, 16-17, 20
Farms, 24, 25-26, 37, 113, 114, 127-128, 135-136, 139-142. *See also* Gardens
Farm Store, 141
Farrar-Mansur House, 124-125, 129
First Church of Christ, 44, 47
Fleming Museum, 146, 148
Fletcher Farm School for the Arts and Crafts, 128-129, 130
Flume, The, 94-95
Flume Visitor Center, 94, 95-96, 99
Flynn Theatre, 147, 148, 149
Fort George, 163, 166
Fox Hunt Farms, 24, 26, 27
Franconia, New Hampshire, 100-105
Franconia Notch, New Hampshire, 94-100
Franconia Notch State Park, 94-97, 99
Franconia-Sugar Hill Ski Touring Complex, 100, 105
Freedom Trail, The, 48-49, 53. *See also* Boston By Foot; Brush Hill Tours
Freeport, Maine, 150-156
Front Beach, 67
Frost Place, The, 100-101, 105

Gardens, 16, 17, 22, 24-25, 44, 61-62, 101, 113, 122, 140, 170-171. *See also* Farms
Gardner-Pingree House, 58
Golden Age Passport, 11
Grace Cottage Hospital Fair Day, 117
Granary, The, 159, 160
Granite Pier Wharf, 68, 70
Granstrom's Fruit Farm, 135-136, 137
Greater Boston Convention and Visitors Bureau, 48, 53
Green Briar Nature Center and Jam Kitchen, 41, 46
Guided tours, 22-23, 36-37, 41, 43, 49-51, 52-53, 57-58, 60, 61, 67, 80, 85-86, 123, 134

Halibut Point Reservation, 68–69, 70
Hamlet Hill Vineyards, 25–26, 27
Handicap access, 12, 46, 47, 62, 82, 83, 99, 100, 124, 130, 143, 149
Handworks Gallery, 167, 171
Hanover, New Hampshire, 106–111
Hanover League of New Hampshire Craftsmen, 109–110, 111
Hapgood Pond Recreation Area, 127, 130
Harman's Cheese and Country Store, 103, 105
Harraseeket Lunch, 154, 155
Harris Foods, Ltd., 32, 33
Hart's Turkey Farm Restaurant, 92, 93
Haystack Mountain School of Crafts, 168–170, 172
Heritage Plantation of Sandwich, 44–45, 47
Hickin's Mountain Mowings Farm and Greenhouses, 113, 118
Hiking, 32, 73–74, 81–82, 95, 97, 117, 123, 142
Historical Society of Windham County, 114, 118
Historic sites, 16, 17–18, 21–24, 34–35, 43–44, 48–53, 57–58, 59–61, 64, 74–75, 84–87, 100–101, 107, 114, 117, 120, 122–123, 124–125, 129, 139–141, 163, 164. *See also* Museums
Holbrook Wildlife Sanctuary, 162
Hood Museum of Art, 19, 108, 111
Hopkins Center, Dartmouth College 107, 111
Horseshoes Tournament, Annual, 117
Housatonic Trading Co./Country Things, 31, 33
House of Seven Gables, 60, 61–62, 63
Hoxie House, 43, 47

Images Cinema, 78, 82

Jim's Dockside, 38–39
John Hancock Observatory, 51–52, 54
John Perkins House, 163, 166
John Ward House, 57
Joseph Cerniglia Winery, 127–128, 130

Kent Falls State Park, 32, 33
Kent Station Square, 31
Kneisel Hall, 167, 171
Kristina's, 158–159, 160

Lafayette Campground, 96, 99
Lawrence's Smokehouse, 115–116, 119

League of New Hampshire Craftsmen, Hanover, 109–110, 111
Ledges Interpretive Trail, 74
Leighton Gallery, 167, 171
Little Art Cinema, 67, 70
L.L. Bean, 150–152, 155
L.L. Bean clinics, 151
L.L. Bean Fly Fishing Schools, 151, 155
L.L. Bean Paddling Lesson, 151
Local transport, 12, 51, 55, 65, 158
Ludlow, Vermont, 129

Maine, 150–172
Maine Maritime Museum, 150, 156–158, 160
Mary's Place, 73, 75
Massachusetts, 40–83
Mast Landing Sanctuary, 153, 155
Meadow House, 170–171, 172
Meredith, New Hampshire, 88–93
Middlebury, Vermont, 131–137
Middlebury College Concert Series, 131–132, 136
Middlebury College Snow Bowl, 132, 136
Millbrook Meadow, 68, 70
Mill Falls Marketplace, 89–90, 93
Molly's Balloon, Ltd., 110, 111
Montshire Museum of Science, 110–111
Morgan Horse Farm, University of Vermont, 135, 136–137
Mount Greylock State Reservation, 81–82
Mount Philo State Park, 142, 143
Museums, 17, 19, 31–32, 36–37, 42–43, 44–45, 50, 55–56, 58–59, 76–77, 82, 90–91, 98–99, 103–104, 107–108, 110–111, 120–121, 134–135, 137–139, 146, 156–158, 163–164
Museum Wharf, 50
Music Mountain, 32, 33
M/V *Southland*, 38, 39

Narragansett, Rhode Island, 34–39
Natural Bridge State Park, 80–81, 83
Nature areas, 12, 18–19, 35, 38, 41, 67, 68–69, 73–74, 81–82, 97, 117, 127, 153, 162, 165. *See also* Parks
New England Ski Museum, 98–99, 99–100
Newfane, Vermont, 112–119
Newfane Antiques Center, 113–114, 118
Newfane Country Store, 115, 119
Newfane Flea Market, 116, 119
Newfane Inn, 114–115, 118
Newfane Store, 115, 119

New Hampshire, 84–111, 122–123, 124
New Hampshire Music Festival Orchestra, 90, 93
Noah's Ark, 102, 105
Nonwalking tours, 12, 38, 49–51, 53, 55, 68, 88–89, 97, 113, 117, 137, 142, 147–148, 158, 161, 162
No-Key, 67–68, 70
Norfolk, Connecticut, 28–33
Norfolk Chamber Music Festival, 32, 33
North Adams, Massachusetts, 76–83
North Adams General Store, 80
North Country Chamber Players, 104–105
Northeast Corner (Connecticut), 21–27

Off-season specials, 7–8, 12, 35–36, 69, 100
Ogden House, 15, 16–17, 20
"Old-fashioned" fun, 12, 45, 89, 114, 135–136, 142
Old Man of the Mountain, 96, 97, 99
Old Meeting House, 164
Old Print Barn, The, 91–92, 93
One-stop attractions, 8–9, 12, 47–70, 76–83, 106–111, 161–166
Otter Creek Café & Bakery, 133–134, 136

Parks, 12, 19, 24, 32, 68, 79–81, 94–97, 116, 117, 142, 153. *See also* Nature areas
Passumpsic Round Barn, 137–138
Peabody Museum of Salem, 55–56, 62
Pedal and Paddle, 72–73, 75
Performing arts, 17, 20, 32, 65–67, 69, 77–78, 90, 104–105, 107, 123, 125–126, 131–132, 146–147, 160, 165, 167
Petty's Pizza, 163, 166
Pickering Wharf, 59, 62
Plainfield Greyhound Park, 26–27
Planning your travels, 6–13
Plymouth, Vermont, 127–130
Plymouth Cheese Corporation, 129
Polly's Pancake Parlor, 102, 105
Pomfret, Connecticut, 21–27
Pomfret Antique World, 25, 27
Pool, The, 95
Pumpkin Festival, 117

Queen of Winnipesaukee, 89, 93

Ralph Myhre Golf Course of Middlebury College, 132, 136
Rhode Island, 34–39

174 / INDEX

Rhode Island Party & Charter Boat Association Fishing Tournament, 38
Rockport, Massachusetts, 63–70
Rockport Art Association, 65–66, 69
Rockport Chamber Music Festival, 66–67, 69–70
Rockport Conservation Commission, 67, 70
Roseland Cottage. *See* Bowen House
Roseland Park, 24, 27
Route 7 (Connecticut), 28–33
Route 30 (Vermont), 112–119
Rowantrees Pottery, 168, 172

Saint-Gaudens National Historic Site, 122–123, 124
Salem, Massachusetts, 54–63
Salem Maritime National Historic Site, 59–60, 62–63
Salem Trolley, 55, 62
Salem Witch Museum, 58–59, 62
Sandwich, Massachusetts, 40–47
Sandwich Glass Museum, 42, 46
Sandwich's Sandwiches, 45–46, 47
Sandy Bay Historical Society, 64, 69
Save the Children Craft Shop, 19–20, 21
Scarborough State Beach, 35, 39
Scenic areas, 21–27, 32–33, 63–76, 84–119, 131–137, 150–156, 161–172
Scott's Covered Bridge, 117
Senior discounts, 10–12, 20, 27, 33, 47, 53, 54, 62, 93, 99, 105, 136, 149, 160
Sewall House, 158
Shaker Village Canterbury, 84–87
Sheffield, Massachusetts, 71–76
Sheffield Pottery, 72, 75
Shelburne, Vermont, 137–143
Shelburne Farms, 139–141, 143
Shelburne House, 140, 143
Shelburne Museum, 137–139, 142–143
Sheldon Museum, 134–135, 136
Shelter Institute, 159, 160
Sherwood Island State Park, 19, 21
Shopping, 19–20, 31, 59, 89–90, 102, 147, 152–153, 167–168. *See also* Crafts; Museums
Silo, The, 30–31, 33
Simple Pleasures of Maine, 164, 166
Sloane-Stanley Museum, The, 31–32, 33
South County Museum, 36–37, 39
South Freeport Marine, 154, 155
Southland, M/V, 38, 39
Spirit of Ethan Allen, 147–148, 149

State of Maine, 161, 162, 165
Sterling and Francine Clark Art Institute, 76–77, 82
Stosh's Ice Cream, 31, 33
St. Paul's Church, 17–18
Sugar Hill, New Hampshire, 100–105
Sugar Hill Historical Museum, 103–104, 105
Sugar Hill Sampler, 102–103, 105
Sun Tavern, 18
Sweet Cecily, 133, 136

Thomas Dexter's Grist Mill, 43–44, 47
Thornton W. Burgess Museum, 41, 42, 46
Ticonderoga, 137, 138
Towers, The, 34–35, 37, 39
Townshend, Vermont, 112–119
Townshend Dam Recreation Area, 117, 119
Townshend Family Park, 116, 119
Townshend Flea Market, 116, 119
Townshend State Park, 117, 119
Trips-at-a-Glance, 13
Turtle Gallery, 167, 171–172

University of Vermont Morgan Horse Farm, 135, 136–137
Upcountry Provisions & Café, 90
USS *Constitution*, 49, 50–51, 53, 54
USS *Constitution* Museum, 51, 53, 54

Vermont, 112–149
Vermont Country Store, 127, 130
Vermont Reds, 147, 149
Vermont State Craft Center at Frog Hollow, 132–133, 136
Vermont State Craft Center at Windsor, 121–122, 124
Vermont Wildflower Farm, 141–142, 143

Water sports, 12, 19, 32, 35, 37–38, 67, 68, 72, 99, 117, 151–152, 153, 154, 165
Webster Cottage, 107, 111
Western Gateway Heritage State Park, 79–80, 83
Weston, Vermont, 124–130
Weston Bowl Mill, 126, 130
Weston Fudge Shop, 127, 130
Weston Playhouse, 125, 130
Westport, Connecticut, 15–21
Westport Country Playhouse, 20, 21
West River Canoe Center, 117, 119
Wilder Barn, 129
Wilder House, 129
Williams Bookstore, 79, 83
Williams College Museum of Art, 77, 82

Williamstown, Massachusetts, 76–83
Williamstown Theatre Festival, 77–78, 82
Wilson Museum, 163–164, 166
Windham County, Historical Society of, 114, 118
Windsor, Vermont, 119–124
Windsor Station Restaurant, 121, 124
Wine Cellar, The, 153, 155
Winnipesaukee Flagship, 88–89, 93
Winnipesaukee Railroad, 89, 93
Winslow Memorial Park, 153, 155
Winterset Designs, 116
Woodbutcher Tools, 159–160
Woodstock, Connecticut, 21–24, 27
Workshops, 29–30, 87, 110, 122, 128–129, 132–133, 164, 168–170. *See also* Classes

Yankee Artisan, 159, 160
Year-round spots, 12, 15–33, 47–63, 71–83, 94–111, 124–136, 156–160
Ye Olde Pepper Companie, 60–61, 62, 63
Yesteryears Doll Museum, 42–43, 46–47
Yuletide Smorgasbord, 69

INDEX / 175

About the Author

A free-lance writer since her graduation from college, Harriet Webster is the author of *Great Family Trips in New England, Coastal Daytrips in New England, Favorite Weekends in New England,* and *Favorite Short Trips in New York State.* She wrote *Winter Book,* a nonfiction children's book, and together with her husband she wrote *18: The Teenage Catalog* and *The Underground Marketplace.*

Her articles have been published in *McCall's, Mademoiselle, Family Circle, Parents Magazine, Working Mother, Better Homes and Gardens, Seventeen, Woman's World, Bride's Magazine,* and *Yankee.* Her travel stories have appeared in *Americana, The Boston Globe, The Christian Science Monitor, Newsday,* and *Boston* magazine. She lives in Gloucester, Massachusetts, with her husband and three sons.